Stay Young

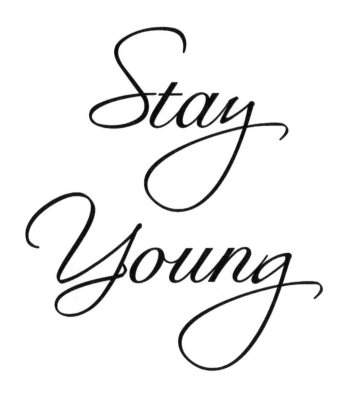

Stay Young

10 Proven Steps to Ultimate Health

by

J. Mark Anderson, MD, DABFM
Walter Gaman, MD, DABFM, FAAFP
Judith K. Gaman, BSHS, CCRC, CMA

George House Publishing

ISBN: 978-0-9840731-0-8
Printed in the United States of America

Dedications

Walter Gaman – I would like to dedicate this book to my family. They are a never ending river of dedication and wondrous events. They are unbelievable.

Mark Anderson – The staff at Executive Medicine of Texas gives unsurpassed service to our patients. I dedicate this book to them for all their hard work.

Judy Gaman – This book is dedicated to my grandfather, John C. Grieve, who lived to be 91 and enjoyed every moment of life. He left a legacy of love and compassion that will last for generations. I hope that everyone can live long and as fulfilled as he did.

To Walter, who inspires me every day and who has kept his promise that there will never be a dull day. You are my rock and I am so happy to share each day with you.

To my children, each one has endured the long hours of distraction that writing a book can cause. I love you and am so proud of you all. No mother could ask for more than you continue to give me, you are wonderful.

Lastly, but most importantly, I dedicate these pages to God who gives me inspiration and strength each day. May His blessings pour upon all who read these pages in an effort to better their life.

Acknowledgements

The names on the cover are only half the story. It takes a team to bring together a book and inspire others. Without the following people, this book would not be the same.

Our sincerest thanks to:

Leah Stovall – Your editing and ideas are always so appreciated. Thank you for your dependability and having such a good heart.

Joy Pike – You are simply amazing and inspiring. Each day we see the wheels turning and your ideas, input, and enthusiasm are contagious.

Sarah Tharnish – Without your daily push of "go write!" this book would never have made it to completion. You are wonderful.

George Pelletier – You are a dear friend and we are blessed to know someone as wonderful as you. Not only are you highly respected by so many, but we think you are one of the most intelligent people we know. We are forever grateful to you for writing the Foreword for this book, and for all the other great things you have done over the years.

Brion Sausser – Thank you so much for the fantastic book design. You are the best in the business!

Contents

Introduction...11

Preamble: A New Time with New Challenges........................15

Step #1: Know Your Family History..............................25

Step #2: Know Your Current Status.............................37

Step #3: Modify Your Eating Habits.............................75

Step#4: Go to the Spa...91

Step #5: Adopt an Exercise Program............................101

Step #6: Get Spiritually Centered................................113

Step #7: Take Control of Your Work and Home Life............119

Step#8: Have Sex Often..129

Step #9: Sleep Your Way to a Younger You....................139

Step #10: Have Fun and Enjoy Life.............................147

Six Month Follow-Up..155

Foreward

Our personal world is dictated by the health of our bodies. Our body is a product of how we treat it and the gene pool we inherited. Should our body feel poorly of a day, we probably will not perform well. Nor are we likely to be as happy as when our bodies are in perfect harmony with our minds and abilities. Age makes it more difficult to maintain harmony. We all eventually need help in our efforts to stay young on the inside so that we can feel young on the outside. This book gives us the guidelines we so desperately need to do just that. Following these steps will give you not only a healthy body, but more confidence in yourself.

The authors are good friends of long standing and my doctors. They have proven themselves by literally saving me, catching medical problems before they became overwhelming. When I started feeling like it was time to slow down, they discovered that my sluggishness was not from getting older, but a medical condition. Once diagnosed and treated, I had a new lease on life and felt 20 years younger. Another time while I was undergoing a thorough physical they discovered a tumor, early enough to be removed successfully and followed by a full recovery. Advanced medical testing becomes the nexus of successful survival as we grow older. Having a physician and medical team that practices state of the art medicine is what saved my life.

Executive Medicine of Texas, where these doctors practice medicine, is one of the best facilities for proactive and preventative medicine in their area of the country. They take time to treat the patient as a whole, not just in reaction to problems and issues. One of the first practices to recognize the importance of in-depth individualized care; they change lives one at a time. For patients like me – that has made all the difference in my world.

Medical testing alone will not save you. We have to work at getting and staying healthy. This means exercise, proper diet and maintaining a positive mental outlook. Again, the pages that follow tell you how to stay young and go into great detail on each step. The book not only explains what to eat, but also tells why – surprisingly generous in that respect – and even what time of the day is best to exercise depending upon your goal.

This is not a professional's text book, but one written for the lay person. Sometimes you read a book where the author is out to impress you with his or her knowledge on the subject matter; which for the average person, makes for tedious reading. This book is for the likes of us who are not medical professionals but want to know the best and most current information on keeping ourselves healthy all in a format that we can follow.

There is a good reason our recent Ex-Presidents have lived so long and been so healthy. They are watched over and receive the proper medical tests on a timely basis. It is this personal care and medical attention that Stay Young: 10 Proven Steps to Ultimate Health details for the rest of us. Follow what is set forth herein and you will live a healthier, longer, and more satisfying life. I know, because I am living proof.

–George A. Pelletier, Santa Fe, New Mexico January 2010

Introduction

In our quest to help people live healthier lives, we have realized the need for clear concise talk on how to stay young while managing the outside stresses of the world. Today, we are faced with having to accomplish more than is humanly possible. Our jobs, families, and society as a whole keep beckoning us to do more and be more.

While the pressure to be everything to everyone is at an all time high, so is the pressure to stay young and beautiful. It is as if two conflicting messages are tugging at the body, spirit, and mind. The challenge to stay healthy and youthful is onerous. Single, married, with or without children, you know the pressures of living in today's society.

We see patients daily that are working endless hours at the office so that they can either achieve financial goals, or catch up to the high debt that they have piled up. Long hours at the office, coupled with the lack of adequate down time, nutrition, or sleep can be a recipe for disaster. While, we understand the need for occasional overtime, or a detour from living and eating healthy, it is important to develop and keep good habits overall. We deceive ourselves when we keep going and plugging along. The truth is we are becoming less and less effective because we don't stop to take care of ourselves.

Think of your body as a car. You can be any car you want to be: a sedan, an SUV, or a high performance sports car. You would never dream of running a car without stopping for gas, changing the oil, or rotating the tires. The car would eventually stop running and become useless. The same is true for our bodies, we have to take the time to take care of ourselves or eventually we will be no good to anyone, including ourselves.

Throughout the pages of this book, we will look at the components of staying young, how you can incorporate these components into your daily routine and make the subtle changes that will elicit a big difference in your overall health. Change is easier when you do it with pure motivation and determination, but it may also be more adoptive if you make changes in stages or "baby steps" each week. For this purpose, each step ends with a few reflective questions that will help take you to the next step by applying the reading to your personal circumstances.

Before you can implement changes, you must first understand your current state of health. We will walk you through a process of discovery, have you document your current status, and set goals for achieving optimal health. By documenting information from your physical exam, your genetic predispositions, your home and work life, and other factors, a clearer picture of what health risks you have will materialize. This will help you develop a plan for change.

First, before you can determine where you want to go, you must have a very clear understanding of where you are. Then set goals that are both measurable and achievable to begin your new health and wellness plan. The step on nutrition will help you evaluate your eating habits and also take you through fad diets to explain why they are not the best bet for getting and keeping you healthy. Each step in the Stay Young process is developed for long-term benefits. This is not a temporary fix, but instead provides you with the tools to make long lasting changes that will increase your quality of life.

We commend you for your positive attitude and search for a better and healthier life. You should be proud of yourself for taking the first steps to make your future brighter and your body and mind younger. As caregivers, we are honored to be part of the process. Now, let's get started!

Preamble:

A New Time with New Challenges

Close your eyes and think back to 1990. Imagine deciding to go out for the day and take a break from it all. Maybe you are dreaming of the golf course, a stroll in the park, or a day at the spa. Whichever it is, the best part of this image is the part about getting "away" from your stressors. It was just a short time ago, but it was a lifetime in terms of technology. Back then, you could actually get away. Cell phones were mostly for emergencies, you didn't have a nagging feeling to check your voicemail, email, Facebook, or any other form of communication. It was just you and your peaceful surroundings.

Current technological advancements have made a world of difference in our lives. Everything is faster and more efficient. For the most part, we can do four or five things while not even having to stop to think about what we are doing. Our minds have become little computers that are mostly on automatic pilot as we buzz through the day. At the end of the day our head hits the pillows in wonderment of "what exactly happened today?"

If you are a busy professional, your day may start with early morning meetings, lots of decision making, voicemail, email, the kids and spouse texting you, and the list goes on and on. The day ends with much of the same thing followed by picking the kids up, driving them to activities like sports, trying to figure out dinner, and then the infamous pillow again.

Even if you are a stay-at-home parent, your days also are filled with chaos. In the effort to get it all done and be everywhere for everyone, there just aren't enough hours in the day. Days turn into weeks, weeks to months, months to years, and then you are left wondering "where did all the time go?"

Taking the time to categorize where all the hours are going is the first step in bringing some sanity into your busy world. Dr. Joyce Myers, a world famous minister, makes a great point when she speaks of the word "busy". It is her opinion the word "busy" should be added to the list of four letter words and should be banned from our every day vocabulary.

If you think about it, we use the word "busy" as a fill-in-the-blank excuse for why we aren't doing the things that are important in our lives. For example, your mother calls and asks why you haven't been around or called. Your excuse – busy. Your child wants you to play with them or help them with home work. You guessed it – busy. You feel tired and in need of rest – oh well, too busy for that too!

It's time that we take control of our lives and stopped being so "busy". Let's periodically go back in time by turning off our cell phones, refusing to check our email, and kicking back and enjoying life every now and again. Call up old friends, meet for coffee, send your parents or other family members a card or flowers just to say "hello". Breath in, breath out, repeat.

All this may seem like fluff and niceties, but there is medical science behind the rational. Overall depression is on the rise and is affecting us all. A Harvard Medical Center study reported that the rate of childhood depression is increasing 23% a year. It is hard to separate the mental health effects from the growing demands on us as individuals. As we have grown accustomed to the fast pace of life, we find it harder and

harder to slow down and relax. Unfortunately, we are raising a genera-
tion that may never know what it feels like to relax. It is up to each of
us to break the cycle and stop the insanity.

Many times our patients come in and say that they took time off
but still don't feel rested. After further questioning, they didn't really
take time off, they simply worked from home or their vacation spot.
Even doing this a few minutes a day can disrupt the brains ability to
relax and decompress. Just because you can check up on things, doesn't
mean that you should. There is a good book out that we recommend
to our patients who just can't seem to get away, *Chained to the Desk: A
Guidebook for Workaholics, Their Partners and Children, and the Clinicians
who Treat Them* by Brian Robinson. If you have a hard time getting away
from work, we strongly suggest that you read it.

Although technology was introduced to help us save time at work
and allow for more family time, the opposite has happened. Today's
American works on average 47.1 hours, with some working up to seventy
hours a week. It has been over seventy-five years since we have seen
work hours this long. Other countries are also following suit, creating
an overworked world.

We will talk more about this later in the book, but vacations are a
time for relaxation and recharging the batteries within our bodies and
spirits. However, they are something that we are failing to take advantage of. At this time, more than ever, you must ignore the cell phone
and computer and refuse to be sucked into the vortex of the 24/7/365
work day. Health without relaxation is impossible.

The Workplace

As time has passed, so has the traditional work environment. Long
gone are the days that we worked outside and then chopped and carried
wood in order to stay warm at home. While our ancestors were subject

to daily manual labor, it came with its benefits. Daily exercise and fresh air are good for our bodies and our mental health. Our ancestors were less likely to stress out over little things, and depression was significantly less prevalent. The body had natural hormones called endorphins that kept people happy as they worked away the day. Schedules also allowed for adequate sleep and relaxation.

The majority of current working environments consist of offices and heavy computer work. Less time is spent doing manual labor and more time is spent in stationary or sitting positions. These sedentary types of jobs come with their own set of health concerns. Below are a list of common health concerns in the work place and how to avoid them:

Eye Strain: Computers can actually cause your eyes to fatigue and affect your vision. You can avoid or lessen eye strain by positioning your computer screen 18-30 inches from your eyes. Also, look away for 20 seconds for every 20 minutes you are on the computer. Do this by focusing on a spot on the wall that is at least 5 feet away.

Back Pain: Looking down at a computer screen or at papers on your desk for long period of time can cause back pain. Be sure to avoid slouching at work by bringing your monitor to eye level. If you do a lot of reading you may want to purchase a stand to bring your papers up to eye level as well. Furthermore, choosing a good ergonomic chair will prevent lower back pain by giving support to overtaxed muscles.

Stress: It seems that stress has become a catch-all phrase that has gained a great amount of popularity in the last couple of decades. The truth is that stress is a common factor in many serious diseases and disorders. Stress has even been linked to the progression of multiple cancers. Some ways to minimize your level of stress is to regulate work hours, take a few 10 minute mental breaks during the day, read something you like during your lunch break, and exercise on a regular basis.

Stress is such a complex and significant health issue, and we will address it again later in great detail.

Vitamin Deficiencies: Working long hours often comes with the side effect of a poor diet. Being inside and away from the sun also adds to the likelihood of disorders such as Vitamin D deficiency, which is linked to cancer, multiple sclerosis, and heart disease. There are many vitamin and mineral deficiencies that are linked to other disease and disorders. These are discussed in greater detail throughout the book.

Depression: In the past few decades we have seen a substantial link between depression and the work place. People used to view their position at work as part of their identity but now it seems that more people see their jobs as a J-O-B, rather than a career. The lack of enthusiasm and enjoyment of work leads to depression. One way to avoid these pitfalls is to go for a walk on your lunch break or try to eat outside of the workplace. A change in scenery will help increase mood and ward off burn-out. An additional way to increase mood and avoid depression is to create a personal space that includes photos from home, colors that you like, and a live plant. Several years back they did a study that showed live plants help decrease stress in the workplace. Workers who had live plants in their work areas seemed happier and stayed employed longer.

Regardless of your current occupation, the pitfalls of the modern workforce include long hours and less down time. If you are lucky enough to work for a corporation that has a gym or wellness program, by all means join it and take steps to help yourself stay healthy. If not, take steps to get healthy by identifying ways to exercise either before or after work.

At Home

The challenges we face at work are coupled with a new way of life at home. Television and computers are showing up in homes across the country in multiple numbers. A single home may have 2-3 computers and a television in just about every room. The focus seems to no longer be about getting outside in the fresh air and meeting neighbors and friends for an evening, but instead most people are opting to stay at home and flip channels or surf the net. Less time is being spent engaging with the members of the family. Take time to turn off the television and computer and enjoy one another.

This lifestyle shift has come with a slew of health pitfalls. Society seems to be on a journey of self-destruction. The good news is that we can change the course and go from self-destruction to self-construction. Below are a few real-life problems that we have seen in our practice over the years, followed by a few tips on how to keep from letting these problems take you over.

Sedentary Lifestyle: This is one of the single most dangerous problems with today's individual. Just because you have the ability to surf through 200 channels a night, doesn't mean that you should. Find ways to get moving so that you can decrease your chances of heart disease, diabetes, and depression. Make an effort to track your daily exercise. If you can, try to exercise outside several times a week. If you live in a climate that doesn't allow for doing so, make sure that you exercise with the television off.

Poor Nutrition: Eating out has become all too common in today's society. When we eat out, we pay less attention to what we eat, and we expose ourselves to additional bacteria and food additives. Make a point of eating at home at least 5 out of 7 days a week. When doing so, pay attention to proportions and the nutritional quality of the food you eat. Nutrition is covered in greater detail later.

Stress: If you have a tendency to bring the office home with you, you will add to the stress in your life. The home should be a place of rest and refuge. Take the time to make your home your castle by creating your personal space. Also, make house rules, like no yelling or arguing. Sure you will have an occasional disagreement, but your home should be a happy place filled with love and respect. Make house rules and follow them. If you are a parent, model the behaviors you want your children to display.

Lack of Sleep: On average, people are getting less sleep than they did in the past. It is not just the amount of sleep that you get, but the quality. Sleep is imperative to healthy brain function and a healthy immune system. You should be sleeping in a cool, dark room for 7-8 hours a night. If you have trouble falling asleep, try journaling at night. This will help you reduce the number of things that run through your head while you try to doze off. If you snore, this could be a caused by sleep apnea, a dangerous condition that can lead to other health problems. Visit your doctor and request a sleep study. When you have the results and recommendations, take steps to increase your sleep quality. If your spouse snores, this could be affecting their health as well as yours. Quality of sleep is just as important as the quantity of sleep.

In this fast paced world, we need to be sure that we are also nurturing our creative side. Creativity exercises the brain and shuts down your stress center. While some people are more creative than others, having a hobby is a great way to reduce stress and increase mood. Whether you enjoy golfing, chess, or collecting things, a hobby is a great way to give yourself a vacation from the realities of life.

Our present culture meets us with new challenges. Throughout the ten steps we will take you through the best ways to meet these challenges and be a healthier, younger you. Take a few minutes to look at the health pitfalls you may be facing at work and at home. Answer the following questions honestly. You are now beginning your journey to better days.

Self Reflection Questions:

On average, how many hours do I spend on the computer each day?
_____ Weekdays _____ Weekend Days _____ Combined Average

Do I have problems with back pain at work? If so, what can I do to correct this issue? (Buy a better chair, raise my computer monitor, do back strengthening exercises, etc.)

_____

_____

_____

How often am I eating out per week? (Include all meals)

_____

_____

_____

How often do I exercise? Is it inside or outside activities? How can I improve this part of my lifestyle?

_____

_____

_____

On a scale of 1-10 (10 being highest) what is my stress level at home? Work?

_____ Home   _____Work

What can I do to improve my stress level?

Home _____

_____

_____

Work _____

_____

_____

What do I like to do as a hobby? Am I taking the time to do this? If not, how can I put my hobby back on my schedule?

_____

_____

_____

Step #1

Know Your Family History

Genetics are often blamed for many of the diseases and disorders that we see today. While many of the problems may be linked to genetics, often it is a combination of environmental and genetic factors. Like baking a cake, the results of a human condition are the make-up of the ingredients, including what you inherent from your parents, genetically, culturally, and environmentally. For example, if you have all the right ingredients, but fail to follow the baking instructions, the cake will either burn or undercook. Likewise, following the cooking instructions, but leaving an ingredient out can cause just as much disappointment with the final product.

In humans, a set of twins could enter the world with the genetic predisposition for lung cancer. One twin may develop the unhealthy habit of cigarette smoking and the other may not. While they both have the genetic risk factors, the environmental factors of smoking may contribute to the absence or presence of the disease. While both of the twins had the predisposition, the one who chose to smoke triggered the cancer to develop.

Research on Cultural or Ethnic Predispositions

Predispositions to particular diseases and disorders is in the infancy stages as we make advancements in medicine, but we do have some data that shows prevalence is associated with both race and culture.

Caucasians are less likely to have diabetes than Latinos and African Americans, but more likely to develop COPD (Chronic Obstructive Pulmonary Disease). African Americans are more likely to develop serious heart conditions, but are less likely to die from liver disease than other races.

Caucasian women have the highest overall risk of breast cancer, except between the ages of 40-50, where African American women have the highest risk. African American women also are more likely to die from the disease, while Chinese American women have the lowest death rate of all breast cancer victims. This is why doctors and other healthcare providers need to assess patients and determine treatment on an individual basis.

While it was once believed that lower survival rates by different races may be due to socioeconomic status and access to health care, a new study suggests otherwise. The 2009 study was funded by the National Cancer Institute and conducted by the Loyola University Health System. A group of 19,457 cancer patients were studied and followed for 10 years after treatment. Treatment and detection of the disease was equivalent across racial boundaries. African Americans were significantly more likely to die from breast, ovarian, and prostate cancer. Other cancers did not show a racial divide. This study suggests that genetic factors play a more significant role than socioeconomic factors in death rates for certain types of cancers.

This same theory could explain why different races have a predisposition or more significant death rate to different diseases. The study did not reveal any information why certain races develop the disease in the first place. This is where genetics, as well as cultural factors come in to play.

Not only by race, but by culture, one can find factors that affect the long term health and wellness of a person, in either a positive or negative way. For example, Asian's are generally healthier and have lower risk for heart disease, cancer, and diabetes. Much of this may be due to their diet. Nutrition is discussed at great length in another section of this book, but understanding the overall impact of nutrition in preventing disease is the first step in changing some of the cultural health divides that populations currently experience.

The statistical data that shows Caucasians to have a higher instance of COPD than any other race, suggests it's due to poor working conditions within factories and mines, along with cigarette smoking that was historically more frequent and started earlier in life. While this data is subjective, it may explain why the gap is narrowing in the current population. Could this be due to improved working conditions and increasingly more parallel smoking patterns? Some suggest so, but others suggest that narrowing gaps have to do with the diluted genetic pool. Either way, this is why medical research is not only fascinating, but necessary.

Many times cultural influences can be as simple as geographical location. Even within the United States, we have a far different diet in the South than in the Northeast. Also, people living on either coast, will be more likely to eat fish, which is high in Omega-3 fatty acids (a cancer fighting nutrient). Even within the same state, people who live in densely populated cities are exposed to more pollutants than those that live in more rural areas.

Overall, personal health is about understanding predispositions, whether they are cultural, ethnical, or genetic and using that information to your advantage. Your personal health code is like a puzzle, each piece makes the bigger picture clearer. Don't fear your differences, instead embrace them and understand them.

Decoding the Genetic Link

It wasn't until recently that we began to understand the complexity of the human body. Through the mapping of the human genome, we are able to identify particular genetic links to diseases and disorders. Biomedical research is now front and center on the stage of medical advancements and every day scientists are unlocking the key to living longer and healthier. This research helps us decide a course of treatment for our patients and increase their life span.

Scientists now predict that each person has 5-10 deadly genetic mutations, but since the mutations may only be from one parent, meaning only half the risk, many of us will be lucky enough to never experience the disease. This is why physicians are so interested in their patient's family history. If a condition is present on both sides of the family, the risk for developing the disease or disorder is significantly higher. Knowing your risk factors and sharing them with your doctor will help in developing a preventative plan of action that looks for problems in their early stages.

How it Works

Each person is born with 46 chromosomes, including 22 pairs of autosomal chromosomes and 2 sex chromosomes. A pair of chromosomes contains one chromosome from each parent. Within each cell in the body there are 6 billion pairs of nucleotides that contain 30,000 individual blueprints that make a human unique. These blueprints tell the body what to look like and how to function.

DNA is very small and is about 2000 times thinner than a strand of hair. There is so much information within the DNA of one's body that if it was taken from each cell, laid end to end it would stretch to the moon and back 130 times. The explanation of DNA that was discovered by James Watson and Frances Crick in 1953 opened a whole new world of medical discoveries and human understanding that has changed medical mindsets forever.

Genes are usually dominant or recessive. The dominant gene is what is expressed in the outward appearance of a person. For example, if a child comes from a mother with red hair and a father with black hair, if the child has black hair, the father's gene was dominant. The child will still have the genotype (coding) for each color, but their phenotype (what is expressed) is black hair.

Recently, scientists have come to understand that genetics are not always dominant or recessive, some traits are polygenic. This means that a number of genes contribute at the same time. This is easily understood in height and skin color, as these are developed as a combined influence by both parents. Actually, there are 6 genes that combine from each parent to determine the skin color. This is why skin color is a mixture of both parents.

It has been proven that polygenic inheritance has been linked to diabetes, hypertension and heart disease. Basically, it is not just a "diabetic" gene, but a combination of genetic differences that lead to diabetes. This disease, like others, is complex in its predisposition and development.

Many times a polygenic disease or disorder is linked to the inability to rid the body of toxins or allergens. Genes are simply bundled in a way that makes the person more susceptible and less likely to deter the disease. This is especially true in some genetically linked cancers.

Additional Research

One study found that people with type O blood have a 40 percent higher incidence of duodenal ulcers than other blood types. It is not necessarily their blood type that causes the higher risk, but rather the sequence of genes that type O blood carriers have. Other factors, combined with gene sequence, lead to a high incidence of this condition.

Every day new research emerges that gives us insight into the role genetics play in our health. In 2007 Canadian and Icelandic researchers concluded that genetics play a significant role in heart disease. Both studies were run independent of each other, but the conclusions were parallel. The comparison of healthy people to people with known heart disease showed a common genetic variant among those with heart disease. Researchers also discovered that those who possess both genes for the variant have a 30-40 percent higher risk of heart disease, while those with one gene drop to 15-20 percent. Most of all, this explains why some are more affected by unhealthy lifestyles than others.

One of the most recent and most advanced studies explaining polygenic diseases was completed in 2009 by a British led group of investigators from the Alzheimer's Research Trust. The study involved scanning 16,000 people, 4,000 of which had Alzheimer's disease. The research determined that while Alzheimer's had originally only been linked to one gene, there was overwhelming evidence that three genes code for Alzheimer's. CLU and CR1, are genes that are linked to preventing the build-up of plaques. PICALM, the third gene, is linked to nerve receptors and memory. The main cause of Alzheimer's is the absence of CLU and CR1. This discovery explaining the complexity of the disease will speed the discovery of cures and management of the disease. As doctors, we live for these types of breakthroughs. Findings like this mean that a cure is on the horizon.

Not all genetically predisposed diseases are caused by defective genes. The absence of genes can lead to life threatening conditions. For example, some cancer is linked to a missing p53 gene. Without p53, the cell lacks the protein that keeps mutated cells, the cells that cause tumors, from dividing.

Genetic Testing

Previously, genetic testing has been limited to newborn screening and fertility issues. However, new research has surfaced that links genetics and pharmaceutical efficacy, therefore explaining why some people respond better to different medications than others. Someday soon, genetic testing may become a routine way of deciding which drugs to prescribe.

Some DNA tests are available to the general public. The tests help us understand a patient's predisposition to a certain disease. Breast cancer testing may be the most popular, but only 5 percent of breast cancers are genetically linked to the current test mutations. A simple test can screen for the BRCA1 and BRCA2 genes in people that have a strong family history of breast cancer. However, the test does not come without additional risks and concerns. If a patient is positive for the genetic mutations, they still may never develop breast cancer, although they have a high risk. This dilemma raises concerns over the over cautious patient who tests positive and requests a double mastectomy.

While mainstream ethical fears remain about exposing personal DNA, scientist are proving that the benefits of knowing your DNA and sharing that information with health care providers may extend your life, or at least make treating medical problems easier and more effective.

The Future

While the idea is in the development stages, Biochips may someday become part of the medical record and everyone will carry a small card in their wallet that will list their mutations. Doctors will be able to scan the card and look for clues to the diagnosis, as well as chose a medication that will work for the individual patient and their condition. Until Biochips are available and in the mainstream of medicine, it is best to make a complete record of your family history and share it with your doctors.

Also, making your family history available to your children may actually save their life some day. A great place to digitally record your family history and save it electronically is at https://familyhistory.hhs.gov. The US Surgeon General has recognized the importance of knowing your family medical background and sharing it with health care providers; therefore, this free service has been set up and is extremely user friendly. Furthermore, none of your information is shared with the government, once you create your history you save it to your personal records. At the end of this section we have also provided a place for you to make notes about your family history.

Summary

There has been years of research, and we are now at the brink of great medical breakthroughs. The historic practice of medicine is evolving into a much more individualized approach. This means that patients, just like you, will play an even more vital role in their care. Knowing your family history is not only important information about the past, it holds valuable clues about your future. You may have to ask other family members, but take the time to record accurate information about your family history – it may just save your life.

On the next page is a list of common diseases, followed by spaces for you to record them if applicable. There may be other diseases and disorders that are not listed here. Be sure to document as much information as possible. Family history can also be recorded on pages 50-56.

Diseases and Disorders:

☐ Alzheimer's	☐ Eczema
☐ Aneurysm	☐ Emphysema
☐ ADD	☐ Endometriosis
☐ ADHD	☐ Fibromyalgia
☐ Anorexia	☐ Graves' Disease
☐ Anxiety	☐ Heart Attack
☐ Arthritis	☐ Hemophilia
☐ Asthma	☐ Kidney Disease
☐ Autoimmune Disease	☐ Leukemia
☐ Bipolar Disorder	☐ Lupus
☐ Bulimia	☐ Macular Degeneration
☐ Cardiovascular Disease	☐ Multiple Sclerosis (MS)
☐ Cancer (specify)	☐ Obesity
☐ Cataracts	☐ Parkinson's Disease
☐ Celiac Disease	☐ Peripheral Vascular Disease
☐ Diabetes	☐ Stroke
☐ Crohn's Disease	☐ Sudden Infant Death Syndrome (SIDS)
☐ Dementia	☐ Thyroid Disease
☐ Depression	☐ Transient Ischemic Attack (TIA)

Relatives:

Relative	Name	Condition(s)
Son		
Son		
Son		

Daughter
Daughter
Daughter
Brother
Brother
Brother
Sister
Sister
Sister
Father
Paternal Grandmother
Paternal Grandfather
Paternal Aunt
Paternal Aunt
Paternal Aunt
Paternal Uncle
Paternal Uncle
Paternal Uncle
Cousin
Cousin
Cousin
Mother
Maternal Grandmother
Maternal Grandfather
Maternal Aunt
Maternal Aunt
Maternal Aunt
Maternal Uncle
Maternal Uncle

Maternal Uncle

Cousin

Cousin

Cousin

Step #2

Know Your Current Status

The term physical exam can be somewhat misleading. Whereas it once only referred to the part of the exam where the physician actually touched the patient to "physically" examine them, it now refers to the history, physical touch, laboratory tests, and any other tests deemed necessary by the physician at the time of exam. In Step #1 we explained the importance of knowing your family history and relaying that information to your health care provider. It is one of many pieces to the puzzle that your doctor will need when determining your current health status and developing a plan of action.

Before we discuss what a good yearly exam entails, let's go over what it is not. There seems to be some confusion in the general population, which has lead many patients to have a false sense of wellness. Here is a list of what a physical exam is NOT:

A physical exam is NOT a pap smear with an OBGYN. This is simply one part of the exam. The heart, lungs, and many other parts of your body must be examined. For example, women are at a greater risk of dying from a heart attack, yet they are often under or misdiagnosed when it comes to heart disease.

A physical exam is NOT a short exam done by your life insurance company. These are highly inadequate and are usually done by a nurse.

There purpose is not diagnostic, but simply to determine your rate and chance for coverage by the insurance company.

A physical exam is NOT what your company offers during a health fair. While these are a nice way to check progress, they are not intended to be diagnostic.

A physical exam is NOT obtainable in a matter of ten minutes. If your doctor doesn't take the time to really get to know you and your history, this is more of a check-up than a true physical exam.

In the defense of many physicians, insurance reimbursements are often very low and doctors must see a large volume of patients to cover their overhead. To ensure that you are getting more time with the doctor you may want to choose one that has a cash paying practice, or will allow you to book extra time at your expense to go over things that your insurance company may not cover. This is especially important if you are symptomatic, or have a strong family history of disease. Please know that doctors, in general, prefer to spend more time with their patients and do a thorough job. Unfortunately, the red tape and expense of running a busy insurance-based practice creates a barrier between the patient and the doctor.

If you can't afford to pay cash for your visit, then be sure to make the most out of your scheduled time with the doctor. Make a list of concerns and bring the list with you. This systematic approach will help you remember what questions you want to ask. Be on time or even early if you will have paper work to fill out. Turn your cell phone off and be ready when the doctor comes in. You would be surprised how many patients are talking on the phone when the doctor comes in to see them. Aside from being rude, this type of distraction only takes time away from you and the other patients that are waiting to be seen.

Not all physical exams are created equal; in an ideal world, everyone would get what is referred to as an "executive physical" and the doctor would spend a matter of hours focusing on just one patient. For the sake of this chapter, we will discuss the ideal exam and what it covers, but know that not every physician can deliver such an exam due to lack of equipment, time, or expertise.

Health History Questionnaire

In preparation for your exam, it is best to fill out a detailed questionnaire that not only gives you insight into your current health status, but gives the doctor a starting point from which to work from. When we are preparing to do an executive physical at our office, we read the patients Health History Questionnaire in detail PRIOR to the patient coming in. We have found that doing so helps us formulate new questions, discuss risk factors, and begin thinking of long term preventative actions that the patient should consider. This is the best way to treat the patient as a whole being, allowing us to find underlying causes and not just treat the symptoms, but instead solve the problem.

Each doctor will have their own version of a questionnaire, but below we have included a thorough health questionnaire that may be helpful. Use it as a guide to collect information on yourself. Each item listed has a significant purpose, so be sure to share the information you gather with your health care provider.

MEDICAL HISTORY QUESTIONNAIRE
GENERAL INFORMATION

Sex: _____ Male _____ Female

Race: _____ White _____ Black _____ Hispanic _____ Asian
_____ American Indian _____ Other (Specify) _____

Place of Birth: _____

Are you presently married or in the past been married?

____Yes ____No

If yes, how many times? _____

Current Marital Status: _____ Single _____ Married

____Divorced _____ Widowed

If currently married, how many years? _____

Number of Children? _____

Highest level of Education: _____

Medical Status

What is your primary reason for your visit today? _____

How many days of work did you miss due to illness last year?_____

How many times did you visit a physician for a medical problem last year? _____

Present Medical Problems:

Problem	Date of Onset	Comments

Review of Systems

General

	Past	Current	Comments
Unexplained weight loss			
Unexplained weight gain			
Unexplained fatigue			

Night sweats			
Unexplained fevers or chills			
Any type of cancer			

Heart and Vascular

	Past	Current	Comments
Chest pain or pressure			
Chest pain with exertion			
Heart attacks			
Irregular heartbeats			
Fainting or lightheadedness			
High blood pressure			
Rheumatic fever			
Leg pain with exercise			
Varicose veins			
Blood clots			
Stroke			
High cholesterol			

Eyes

	Past	Current	Comments
Decrease in vision Date of last eye exam ____/____/____			
Double vision			
Glaucoma			
Color Blindness			
Cataracts			
Serious injury to eye			

Eye correction surgery Date __/__/__			

Ear Nose Throat

	Past	Current	Comments
Hearing Loss			
Prolonged exposure to loud noises			
Ringing in ears			
Chronic ear infections			
Ruptured eardrum			
Snoring			
Sinus problems			
Allergies			
Polyp on vocal cords			
Hoarseness			

Endocrine

	Past	Current	Comments
Thyroid disease			
High blood sugar			
Diabetes			

Pulmonary

	Past	Current	Comments
Chronic cough or phlegm			
Wheezing			
Asthma			
Tuberculosis			
Chronic Bronchitis			

Pneumonia			
Emphysema			
Blood clot in lung			
Coughing up blood			
Unexplained shortness of breath			

Gastrointestinal

	Past	Current	Comments
Fatty food intolerance			
Ulcer disease			
Heartburn			
Vomiting blood			
Gallbladder trouble			
Abdominal pain			
Liver problems			
Frequent diarrhea			
Lactose intolerance			
Blood in stool			
Tarry black stool			
Hemorrhoids			
Colon Polyps			
Constipation			

Genitourinary

	Past	Current	Comments
Sexual transmitted diseases			
Sexual problems			
Decreased sex drive			
Impotence (men only)			

HIV Positive/AIDS			
Blood in urine			
Burning or pain in urination			
Recurrent kidney or bladder infection			
Difficulty urinating			
Prostate problems (men only)			
Awaking at night to urinate			
Kidney stones			

Bone and Joint

	Past	Current	Comments
Joint or muscle pain			
Low back pain			
Swollen or stiff joints			
Arthritis			
Gout			
Osteoporosis or decreased bone mass			

Neuropsychiatric

	Past	Current	Comments
Loss of consciousness			
Vertigo			
Seizures or Epilepsy			
Frequent headaches			
Nervous disorder			
Numbness or tingling of arms, face or legs			
Difficulty sleeping			

Attention deficit disorder			
Depression			
Anxiety			
Thoughts of Suicide			
Psychiatric or Psychological counseling			

Hematology

	Past	Current	Comments
Anemia			
Bleeding disorders			
Enlarged lymph nodes			
Any blood transfusion			

Dermatology

	Past	Current	Comments
Skin rash			
Shingles (Herpes zoster)			
Skin Cancer			
Sores on skin that will not heal			
Unusual Moles			
Breast lumps			
Mouth sores			
Skin fungus			
Nail fungus			
Psoriasis			
Vitiligo (white patches)			

Immunizations

Have you had a tetanus booster in the last 10 years?____Yes____No

Do you get yearly flu vaccines?___Yes ___No

Have you had a pneumonia vaccine?___Yes ___No *(Pneumovax)*

Have you completed a hepatitis A vaccine series?___Yes ___No

(2 vaccines given in six months)

Have you completed a hepatitis B vaccine series?___Yes ___No

(3 vaccines given in six months)

Have you had any other recent immunizations?___Yes ___No

(measles/mumps/rubella booster, polio, typhoid, yellow fever, Lyme disease) please indicate

Do you frequently travel to any of these areas?___Yes ___No

If yes, please circle areas of travel.

(Central/South America   Asia   Middle East   India   Africa)

Have you had a tuberculosis skin test?___Yes ___No

   If yes, was it negative?___Yes ___No

Medication and Vitamin Supplements

Medication	Dosage	Doses	Year Started	Year Stopped

List all current medications including aspirin, oral contraceptives, over-the-counter medications, vitamins, diet supplements, injectable medication, etc.

List all past hormone treatment including estrogen, progesterone, natural estrogen, testosterone, oral contraceptives, etc. above.

Drug Allergies

Are you aware of any allergic reactions to any medications?

___Yes ___No

If so, list medication and reaction to it:

Medication _____

Type of allergic reaction _____

Medication _____

Type of allergic reaction _____

Medication _____

Type of allergic reaction _____

Have you ever had a severe allergic reaction to anything else such as foods, animals or insects or xray dye?___Yes ___No

Gynecological history

When was your last menstrual period? ____/____/____

                                            Month Day Year

When was your last pelvic examination? ____/____/____

                                            Month Day Year

Was the pelvic examination abnormal ___Yes ___No

Are you pregnant?___Yes ___No

Number of pregnancies? _____

Number of live births? _____

Your age at birth of first child? _____

Did you breast feed 3 months or longer? _____

At what age did you begin having menstrual periods? _____

Have you had your uterus removed?___Yes ___No

Have you had your cervix removed?___Yes ___No

Have you had both ovaries removed?___Yes ___No

If yes, at what age? _____

Have you missed your period for 3 months or longer? (excluding pregnancy) ___Yes ___No

Have you gone through menopause (absence of period for 12 months)? ___Yes ___No

Breast Health

When was your last breast examination by a physician?
____/____/____

Month Day Year

Do you examine breasts for lumps each month?___Yes ___No

Are you aware of any breast lumps? ___Yes ___No

Do you have any nipple discharge or bleeding? ___Yes ___No

Have you ever had a mammography performed? ___Yes ___No

If yes, date? _____ Was it abnormal? ___Yes ___No

Have you ever had a breast biopsy? ___Yes ___No

Have you ever had any other breast surgery? ___Yes ___No

Type? _____

Past Medical History

Significant past illnesses as a child or adult:

Illness	Year	Comments

Past Surgery

Type of Surgery	Year	Comments

Radiation Treatment

Area of Radiation	Year	Comments

Diagnostic Studies

Test	Year	Comments

ECG (Electrocardiogram)   _____

Treadmill stress test   _____

Nuclear heart scan   _____

Echocardiogram   _____

Heart catheterization   _____

Upper GI series   _____

Upper endoscopy   _____

Barium Enema   _____

Flex Sig   _____

Colonoscopy   _____

Bone Density   _____

Other   _____

Family Medical History

	Age		Age
	Only if Living		At Death
Father	_____		_____

Health Problems (Mark all that apply)

☐ Heart attacks, coronary bypass, angioplasty, or angina under age 50 (circle problem)

☐ Stroke

☐ High blood pressure

☐ Heart attacks, coronary bypass, angioplasty, or angina under age 50 – 65 (circle problem)

☐ High cholesterol or triglycerides

☐ Diabetes

☐ Colon Cancer

- ☐ Lung Cancer
- ☐ Osteoporosis
- ☐ Breast Cancer
- ☐ Other Cancer

	Age Only if Living	Age At Death
Mother	_____	_____

Health Problems (Mark all that apply)

- ☐ Heart attacks, coronary bypass, angioplasty, or angina under age 50 (circle problem)
- ☐ Stroke
- ☐ High blood pressure
- ☐ Heart attacks, coronary bypass, angioplasty, or angina under age 50 – 65 (circle problem)
- ☐ High cholesterol or triglycerides
- ☐ Diabetes
- ☐ Colon Cancer
- ☐ Lung Cancer
- ☐ Osteoporosis
- ☐ Breast Cancer
- ☐ Other Cancer

Brothers or Sisters (Provide information for each sibling)

	Age Only if Living		Age At Death
Male	_____	Female	_____

Health Problems (Mark all that apply)

- ☐ Heart attacks, coronary bypass, angioplasty, or angina under age 50 (circle problem)
- ☐ Stroke
- ☐ High blood pressure
- ☐ Heart attacks, coronary bypass, angioplasty, or angina under age 50 – 65 (circle problem)
- ☐ High cholesterol or triglycerides
- ☐ Diabetes
- ☐ Colon Cancer
- ☐ Lung Cancer
- ☐ Osteoporosis
- ☐ Breast Cancer
- ☐ Other Cancer

Brothers or Sisters (Provide information for each sibling)

	Age Only if Living		Age At Death
Male	_____	Female	_____

Health Problems (Mark all that apply)

- ☐ Heart attacks, coronary bypass, angioplasty, or angina under age 50 (circle problem)
- ☐ Stroke
- ☐ High blood pressure
- ☐ Heart attacks, coronary bypass, angioplasty, or angina under age 50 – 65 (circle problem)
- ☐ High cholesterol or triglycerides
- ☐ Diabetes

- ☐ Colon Cancer
- ☐ Lung Cancer
- ☐ Osteoporosis
- ☐ Breast Cancer
- ☐ Other Cancer

Brothers or Sisters (Provide information for each sibling)

	Age		Age
	Only if Living		At Death
Male	_____	Female	_____

Health Problems (Mark all that apply)

- ☐ Heart attacks, coronary bypass, angioplasty, or angina under age 50 (circle problem)
- ☐ Stroke
- ☐ High blood pressure
- ☐ Heart attacks, coronary bypass, angioplasty, or angina under age 50 – 65 (circle problem)
- ☐ High cholesterol or triglycerides
- ☐ Diabetes
- ☐ Colon Cancer
- ☐ Lung Cancer
- ☐ Osteoporosis
- ☐ Breast Cancer
- ☐ Other Cancer

Brothers or Sisters (Provide information for each sibling)

	Age		Age
	Only if Living		At Death
Male	_____	Female	_____

Health Problems (Mark all that apply)

☐ Heart attacks, coronary bypass, angioplasty, or angina under age 50 (circle problem)

☐ Stroke

☐ High blood pressure

☐ Heart attacks, coronary bypass, angioplasty, or angina under age 50 – 65 (circle problem)

☐ High cholesterol or triglycerides

☐ Diabetes

☐ Colon Cancer

☐ Lung Cancer

☐ Osteoporosis

☐ Breast Cancer

☐ Other Cancer

Brothers or Sisters (Provide information for each sibling)

	Age		Age
	Only if Living		At Death
Male	_____	Female	_____

Health Problems (Mark all that apply)

☐ Heart attacks, coronary bypass, angioplasty, or angina under age 50 (circle problem)

☐ Stroke

☐ High blood pressure

☐ Heart attacks, coronary bypass, angioplasty, or angina under age 50 – 65 (circle problem)

☐ High cholesterol or triglycerides

☐ Diabetes

- ☐ Colon Cancer
- ☐ Lung Cancer
- ☐ Osteoporosis
- ☐ Breast Cancer
- ☐ Other Cancer

Brothers or Sisters (Provide information for each sibling)

	Age Only if Living		Age At Death
Male	_____	Female	_____

Health Problems (Mark all that apply)

- ☐ Heart attacks, coronary bypass, angioplasty, or angina under age 50 (circle problem)
- ☐ Stroke
- ☐ High blood pressure
- ☐ Heart attacks, coronary bypass, angioplasty, or angina under age 50 – 65 (circle problem)
- ☐ High cholesterol or triglycerides
- ☐ Diabetes
- ☐ Colon Cancer
- ☐ Lung Cancer
- ☐ Osteoporosis
- ☐ Breast Cancer
- ☐ Other Cancer

Brothers or Sisters (Provide information for each sibling)

	Age Only if Living		Age At Death
Male	_____	Female	_____

Health Problems (Mark all that apply)

- ☐ Heart attacks, coronary bypass, angioplasty, or angina under age 50 (circle problem)
- ☐ Stroke
- ☐ High blood pressure
- ☐ Heart attacks, coronary bypass, angioplasty, or angina under age 50 – 65 (circle problem)
- ☐ High cholesterol or triglycerides
- ☐ Diabetes
- ☐ Colon Cancer
- ☐ Lung Cancer
- ☐ Osteoporosis
- ☐ Breast Cancer
- ☐ Other Cancer

Children

	Age Only if Living		Age At Death
Male	_____	Female	_____
Male	_____	Female	_____
Male	_____	Female	_____
Male	_____	Female	_____

Personal Habits

Tobacco

Do you currently use tobacco? _____Yes _____ No

    Cigarettes, how many per day? _____

    What year did you start? _____

    Cigars, how many per day? _____

    What year did you start? _____

    Pipe, how many per day? _____

    What year did you start? _____

    Smokeless tobacco per day? _____

    What year did you start? _____

Have you ever used tobacco? ____Yes ____No

	How many per day	Year Started	Year Stopped	Comments
Cigarettes				
Cigars				
Pipe				
Smokeless Tobacco				

Are you exposed to secondhand smoke? ____Yes ____No

Alcohol

Do you drink alcoholic beverages?____Yes ____No

If yes, how many drinks per week?

Beer (12 oz) _____ Wine (5 oz) _____ Hard Liquor (1.5 oz) _____

Have you used alcohol in the past but quit?____Yes ____No

Do you have or have you ever had problems with excessive alcohol use? ____Yes ____No

If you drink alcoholic beverages...

Have you ever felt you ought to cut down on your drinking?

____Yes ____No

Have people annoyed you by criticizing you drinking?

____Yes ____No

Have you ever felt bad or guilty about your drinking?

____Yes ____No

Have you ever had a drink first thing in the morning to steady your nerves or to get over a hangover?

____Yes ____No

Has your drinking ever affected your job or ability to work?

____Yes ____No

Have you been arrested for driving while intoxicated or under the influence of alcohol?

____Yes ____No

Drugs

Have you ever used or do you currently use recreational drugs?

____Yes ____No

If yes, how often and what type? _____

_____

Weight

What do you consider a good weight for yourself?_____Pounds

What was your highest weight after age 18 (excluding pregnancy)?_____Pounds

At what age? _____

What was your lowest weight after age 18?_____Pounds

At what age? _____

What was your weight at age 21?_____Pounds

Weight loss history: How many times would you estimate you have lost the number of pounds shown below?

	5lbs	10lbs	20lbs	30lbs	50lbs	80lbs	100lbs
Number of times							

Diet

Are you currently on any diet or dietary restriction?___Yes ___No
___ Low Fat ___ Low Salt ___ High Fiber ___ Low Cholesterol
___ Low Calorie___ Other:_____

Meals

In an average week, how many meals do you eat out of 21?_____

Beverages

Give the number of servings that you consume in an average week:

Glasses of Water _____ Milk (8oz) _____ Milk 2% (8oz) _____

Cups of Coffee _____ Regular _____ Decaf

Cups of Tea _____ Regular _____ Decaf

Soft Drinks (12oz) _____ Regular _____ Sugar Free

How many of the above contain Caffeine? _____

Exercise

Do you participate in any type of exercise?___Yes ___No

How many days per week do you exercise on average?_____

Aerobic Activities

Walking ___Yes ___No

How many workouts per week? _____

Average duration? _____ Minutes

How many miles per workout? _____

Average time per mile? _____

Jogging or Running ___Yes ___No

How many workouts per week? _____
Average duration? _____ Minutes

How many miles per workout? _____

Average time per mile? _____

Treadmill (Walking or Running) ___Yes ___No

How many workouts per week? _____
Average duration? _____ Minutes

Speed? _____ Grade _____ Heart Rate _____

Bicycling ___Yes ___No

How many workouts per week? _____
Average duration? _____ Minutes

How many miles per workout? _____

Average time per mile? _____

Stationary Bike ___Yes ___No

How many workouts per week? _____

Average duration? _____ Minutes

How many miles per workout? _____ Heart Rate? _____

Swimming Laps ___Yes ___No

How many workouts per week? _____
Average duration? _____ Minutes

How many miles per workout? _____

Months per Year? _____

Aerobic Dance or Floor Exercise ___Yes ___No

How many workouts per week? _____
Average duration? _____ Minutes

Heart Rate _____

Vigorous Sports (Racquetball, Basketball, etc) ___Yes ___No

Specify:_____

How often per week? _____Average duration? _____ Minutes

What exercise equipment, if any, do you own?_____

To what do you have access to?_____

Muscle Strengthening Activities

Are you currently involved in a muscle strengthening program?
___Yes ___No

___Calisthenics ___Free Weights ___Weight Machines ___

Other: _____

How many days per week do you do these exercises?

_____Average duration? _____Minutes

How long have you been involved in this routine?

_____Years _____Months _____Weeks

Which of the following best describes your muscle strengthening routine?

Upper Body	Lower Body
__Low weights & low reps (<12 reps)	__Low weights & low reps (<12 reps)
__Low weights & high reps (>12 reps)	__Low weights & high reps (>12 reps)
__High weights & low reps (<12 reps)	__High weights & low reps (<12 reps)
__High weights & high reps (>12 reps)	__High weights & high reps (>12 reps)

Flexibility Activities

Are you currently in exercises to maintain or improve your joint flexibility?__Yes__No

What type of exercise? ____Stretching ____Calisthenics ____

Exercise Class ____Yoga

How many days per week do you do these exercises? _____

Duration? _____ Minutes

How long have you been involved in this routine? _____Years _____ Months

Stress and Emotional Factors

How stressful do you consider your home life to be?

_____ Low   _____ Moderate   _____ High

How stressful do you consider your occupation to be?

_____ Low   _____ Moderate   _____ High

How would you classify yourself on the following tension and anxiety scale?

____ No tension, very relaxed

____Slight tension

___Moderate tension

___ High tension

___ Very tense "High-Strung"

What is your greatest source of worry or concern at present?

___ Marriage

___ Family

___ Job

___ Finances

___ Health

___Other

How well do you feel you manage your stress?

___ Not well most of the time

___ Fairly well most of the time

___ Very well most of the time

Do stress and tension in your life seem to cause you to have any of the following symptoms? (Mark all that apply)

___ General irritability or impatience

___ Headaches

___ Abdominal discomfort

___ Sleeplessness ___ Fatigue ___ Other:_____

How often do you use medications, alcohol, or other substances to help you relieve stress and relax?

___ Frequently (Several times a week)

___ Seldom (Once or twice a month)

___ Occasionally (Once or twice a week)

___ Almost never

Please rate your general emotional outlook on life on the following scale:

___ Often Very Depressed

____ Generally Sad

____ Happy and Sad Equal Amount

____ Generally Happy

____ Usually Very Happy and Optimistic

How do you rate your overall health?

____ Poor   ____ Fair   ____ Good   ____ Excellent

Please indicate how often you have felt this way during the past week:

Were you bothered by things that usually don't bother you?

____ 5-7 days ____ 3-4 days   ____ 1-2 days   ____ less than 1 day

Did you have trouble keeping your mind on what you were doing?

____ 5-7 days ____ 3-4 days   ____ 1-2 days   ____ less than 1 day

Did you feel depressed?

____ 5-7 days ____ 3-4 days   ____ 1-2 days   ____ less than 1 day

Did you feel that everything you did was an effort?

____ 5-7 days ____ 3-4 days   ____ 1-2 days   ____ less than 1 day

Did you feel hopeful about the future?

____ 5-7 days ____ 3-4 days   ____ 1-2 days   ____ less than 1 day

Did you feel fearful?

____ 5-7 days ____ 3-4 days   ____ 1-2 days   ____ less than 1 day

Was your sleep restless?

____ 5-7 days ____ 3-4 days   ____ 1-2 days   ____ less than 1 day

Were you happy?

____ 5-7 days ____ 3-4 days   ____ 1-2 days   ____ less than 1 day

Did you feel lonely?

____ 5-7 days ____ 3-4 days   ____ 1-2 days   ____ less than 1 day

Did you feel you could not get "going"?

____ 5-7 days ____ 3-4 days ____ 1-2 days ____ less than 1 day

Lifestyle Risk Evaluation

Do you live in a home without a smoke alarm?

____ Yes ____ No

Do you live in a home without a fire extinguisher?

____ Yes ____ No

Do any household members use alcohol to excess or illegal drugs?

____ Yes ____ No

Do you ever drive or ride in a car without using a seat belt?

____ Yes ____ No

Does anger occasionally affect your driving?

____ Yes ____ No

Have you received any speeding tickets or warnings in the past year?

____ Yes ____ No

Do you ever drive while feeling the effects of alcohol?

____ Yes ____ No

Do you have any hobbies that involve high risk such as racecars, motorcycles or parachuting?

____ Yes ____ No

All of the questions above help us understand your overall health status and health risks.

Laboratory Tests

There are some basic blood tests that are included in most physi-

cal exams, and then there are several advanced tests that can be done for more specific reasons. Below you will find charts that list the basic and advanced tests that are most commonly associated with an exam. The list is not all-inclusive and many other helpful tests are available if deemed necessary by your health care provider.

Basic Labs

Most physical exams will include some basic blood tests. These tests give the health care provider an overview of your general health status. They are designed to look for common diseases and disorders, by identifying abnormalities. Basic lab tests identify a number of issues, but are often just clues to tell the physician which areas of health need to be examined further.

The Complete Metabolic Panel (CMP), Complete Blood Count (CBC), and Urinalysis (UA) are part of all physical exams. Most exams will also include a Sedimentation Rate, Cardio CRP, Lipid Panel, Pap Smear, Thyroid (TSH), Occult Blood Test, and PSA. Below is a breakdown of these laboratory tests.

CMP (Comprehensive Metabolic Panel)	
Glucose	Blood Sugar level
Urea Nitrogen (BUN)	Kidney Function
Creatinine	Kidney Function
EGFR (Estimated Glomerular Filtration Rate)	Kidney Function
BUN/Creatinine Ratio	Kidney Function
Sodium	Electrolyte Level
Potassium	Electrolyte Level
Chloride	Electrolyte Level
Carbon Dioxide	Venous Blood Gas Level
Calcium	Mineral Level
Total Protein	
Albumin	Liver and Kidney Function, Nutritional Status

Globulin	Immune Function
Albumin/Globulin Ratio	Help Reveal Cause of Protein Imbalance
Total Bilirubin	Liver Function
Alkaline Phosphotase	Liver Function
AST or SGOT	Liver Function
ALT or SGPT	Liver Function
CBC (Complete Blood Count)	
White Blood Cell Count (WBC)	Screens for Infection and Leukemia
Red Blood Cell Count (RBC)	Screens for Anemia and Hematological Disorders
Hemoglobin/Hematocrit	Screens for Anemia and Hematological Disorders
Mean Corpuscular Hemoglobin (MCH)	Size of Red Blood Cells, Screens for Various Diseases
MCH Concentration (MCHC)	Concentration of MCH, Screens for Various Diseases
Red Blood Cell Distribution Width (RDW)	Size of Red Blood Cells, Screens for Various Diseases
Hemoglobin/Hematocrit	
Mean Corpuscular Hemoglobin (MCH)	
MCH Concentration (MCHC)	
Red Blood Cell Distribution Width (RDW)	
Platelet Count	
Absolute and Percentages of the following:	
Neutrophils, lymphocytes, Monocytes, Eosinophils, Basophils	This is a dynamic population that varies from day to day depending on current health status. Increases in different areas are associated with some acute and chronic conditions
Urinalysis	
Color and Appearance	Infection and Kidney Function
Specific Gravity	Hydration Level
PH	Acidity or Alkalinity
Ketones	Metabolism
Protein	Infection and Kidney Function
Nitrites	Infection
Urobilinogen	Liver Function
Bilirubin	Liver Function
Red Blood Cells (RBC)	Blood in Urine

White Blood Cells (WBC)	Infection
Leukocyte Estrace	Infection
Other Basic Tests	
Cardio C-Reactive Protein (Cardio CRP)	Cardiac Blockages
Erythrocyte Sedimentation Rate (ESR)	Inflammation (general)
Lipid Panel	
Triglycerides	Fats Causing Heart Disease
Total Cholesterol	Includes LDL and HDL
Low Density Lipoprotein (LDL)	"Bad" Cholesterol
High Density Lipoprotein (HDL)	"Good" Cholesterol
Stool for Occult Blood *This should not take the place of a colonoscopy and is only an initial screening tool. By using an Immunochemical Fecal Occult Blood (ultra sensitive) test, false positives can be avoided.	
Cardiac Testing (Advanced)	
Advanced Lipid Panel	
Total Cholesterol, LDL - C Direct, HDL-C Direct, VLDL-C Direct,	
Triglycerides Direct, Total Non-HDL-C, Total APOB100 Calculated,	
LP(a) Cholesterol, IDL-C, Real- LDL-C, Sum Total LDL-C, Real LDL	
Size Pattern: A, A/B, B, Remnant Lipo, Subclass Information:	
HDL-2 (large and buoyant), HDL-3 (small, dense), VLDL-3 (Remnant Lipo)	
*This test allows us to look at particle size and density. We now know that the normal lipid panel does not yield enough information to assess cardiac risk. With the advanced lipid panel doctors can get a better picture of a patient's lipid profile and determine if and how to treat.	
C-Apolipoprotein A1	Cardiac Risk Indicator
C-Apolipoprotein A1	Cardiac Risk Indicator
B Type Natriuretic Peptide (BNP)	Screens for Heart Failure

Homocystine Level	Progression of Known Heart Disease
Cancer Screening	
CA 125	Ovarian Cancer
CEA	Colon Cancer
PSA	Prostate
BRAC1, BRAC2	Breast
Thin Prep® with HPV	Cervical
Note: These tests are for risk factors only and do not indicate a positive cancer diagnosis. Further testing is required if any of the above tests are positive.	
Hormone Levels	
Follicle Stimulating Hormone (FSH	Infertility, Pituitary, and Menopause
Estrogen	Infertility, and Menopause Markers
Progesterone	Infertility, Diagnostic Tool for Abnormal Uterine Bleeding
Luteinizing Hormone (LH)	Pituitary and Hypothalamic Function, Ovarian and Testicular Cancer
Testosterone	Pituitary and Hypothalamic Function, Testicular Tumors, Impotence
Note: Hormone levels are important in BOTH men and women. They provide the necessary balance for strong bones, cardiac health, and mental clarity.	
Diabetic Testing	
Glucose	Basic Screening
Glycosolated Hemoglobin (Hemoglobin A1C)	Long Term Measure of Glucose Levels
Glucose Tolerance Test	Screens for Diabetes and Hypoglycemia
PreDx (Diabetic Risk Test)	Risk for Developing Diabetes in the next 5 years
Other Important Lab Tests	
Vitamin D Level	Vitamin D Deficiency
Ferritin	Total body Iron
Folic Acid Level	Folic Acid Deficiency/Anemia
GGT	Liver Disease and Inflammation
HIV	Autoimmune Disease

Syphilis	Sexually Transmitted Disease
Chlamydia	Sexually Transmitted Disease
Gonorrhea	Sexually Transmitted Disease
Hepatitis Panel	Screens for Active and Past Disease, and Immunity Levels
Hepatitis A	Liver Disease, Acute, Passed by Food and Direct Contact
Hepatitis B	Liver Disease, Acute and Chronic, Passes by Body Fluid
Hepatitis C	Liver Disease, Chronic, Passed by Body Fluids
Imaging (X-Ray, CT, and Nuclear)	
Chest X-Ray	Basic Test with Minimal information about the Internal Organs Viewed
Full Body CT	
CT of Chest	Screens for Lung Tumors (pulmonary nodules), Organ Inflammation, Cancer
CT of Abdomen	Screens for Tumors especially in the Liver and Kidneys, Gallbladder Disease
CT of Pelvis	Screens for Tumors in the Pelvic Area - Especially Reproductive Organs
CTA	Looks for Calcium in the Coronary Arteries, Provides Cardiac Risk Factors
Virtual Colonoscopy	Uses 3D Reconstruction through CT to Provide Screening for Colon Cancer*
*Note: Virtual Colonoscopy has less side effects than traditional optical colonoscopies. Some software has been proven to be just as if not better than optical colonoscopy. However, if a patient has a history of polyps, a traditional optical colonoscopy may be indicated for polyp removal.	
Bone Density Test	Screens for Osteoporosis
Thallium Stress Test	Scan Added to the Traditional Stress Test for Greater Accuracy*

Note: This is indicated in patients with a strong family history or other risk factors for heart disease.	
Other Important Screening Tests	
Fitness Assessment	Test for Strength and Flexibility
Lifestyle Assessment	Screens for Health Risk Factors
Vision Screen	Eye Sight Check
Color Vision Screen	Early Detection of Macular Degeneration
Nasolaryngoscopy	Vocal Cord Cancer Screening

Piecing it All Together

All of the tests included in the physical exam are clues to help your physician determine your health status. By knowing your status, they can provide a detailed plan to help you live a longer and healthier life. Remember, it is the responsibility of the patient to inform the doctor of all past medical issues and all current symptoms. Do not assume that your health care provider knows what you need. Be proactive and provide as much information as you can. It is a team effort between the patient and the doctor and communication is vital to living a long life and staying healthy.

Record the findings from your physical exam to the following charts.

Be sure to list any abnormal values in your lab work.

Physical Exam

Ears	☐ Normal	☐ Abnormal	_____
Eyes	☐ Normal	☐ Abnormal	_____
Nose	☐ Normal	☐ Abnormal	_____
Throat	☐ Normal	☐ Abnormal	_____
Skin	☐ Normal	☐ Abnormal	_____
Heart	☐ Normal	☐ Abnormal	_____
Lungs	☐ Normal	☐ Abnormal	_____
Extremities	☐ Normal	☐ Abnormal	_____
Abdomen	☐ Normal	☐ Abnormal	_____
Bowel Habits	☐ Normal	☐ Abnormal	_____
Labs:			
CBC	☐ Normal	☐ Abnormal	_____
CMP	☐ Normal	☐ Abnormal	_____
Cholesterol	☐ Normal	☐ Abnormal	_____
Triglycerides	☐ Normal	☐ Abnormal	_____
Other	☐ Normal	☐ Abnormal	_____

Take a moment to record the tests you had and the date so that you can reference them later.

Tests:

Bone Density	☐ Done	☐ Not Done	_____
Chest x-ray	☐ Done	☐ Not Done	_____
CT of the Abdomen	☐ Done	☐ Not Done	_____
CT of the Chest	☐ Done	☐ Not Done	_____
CT of the Pelvis	☐ Done	☐ Not Done	_____
EKG	☐ Done	☐ Not Done	_____
Fitness Assessment	☐ Done	☐ Not Done	_____
Laboratory tests (blood and urine)	☐ Done	☐ Not Done	_____
Mammogram	☐ Done	☐ Not Done	_____
Nasolaryngoscopy	☐ Done	☐ Not Done	_____

Pap smear	☐ Done	☐ Not Done	_____
Stress Test	☐ Done	☐ Not Done	_____
Thallium Stress Test	☐ Done	☐ Not Done	_____
Vision Screen	☐ Done	☐ Not Done	_____
Vision Screen (color)	☐ Done	☐ Not Done	_____
Other	☐ Done	☐ Not Done	_____

List your current height and weight below:

Height _____

Weight _____

View the chart below and record your Body Mass Index (BMI)

Current BMI _____

Weight in Pounds

Height	120	130	140	150	160	170	180	190	200	210	220	230	240	250
4'6	29	31	34	36	39	41	43	46	48	51	53	56	58	60
4'8	27	29	31	34	36	38	40	43	45	47	49	52	54	56
4'10	25	27	29	31	34	36	38	40	42	44	46	48	50	52
5'0	23	25	27	29	31	33	35	37	39	41	43	45	47	49
5'2	22	24	26	27	29	31	33	35	37	38	40	42	44	46
5'4	21	22	24	26	28	29	31	33	34	36	38	40	41	43
5'6	19	21	23	24	26	27	29	31	32	34	36	37	39	40
5'8	18	20	21	23	24	26	27	29	30	32	34	35	37	38
5'10	17	19	20	22	23	24	26	27	29	30	32	33	35	36
6'0	16	18	19	20	22	23	24	26	27	28	30	31	33	34
6'2	15	17	18	19	21	22	23	24	26	27	28	30	31	32
6'4	15	16	17	18	20	21	22	23	24	26	27	28	29	30
6'6	14	15	16	17	19	20	21	22	23	24	25	27	28	29
6'8	13	14	15	17	18	19	20	21	22	23	24	25	26	28

Height in Feet and Inches

■ Healthy Weight   ■ Overweight   ■ Obese

Note: This chart is for adults aged 20 years and older. Source: U.S. Surgeon General

Step #3

Modify Your Eating Habits

For years people have all been told "you are what you eat", a true statement that is now haunting many as they enter the middle years of life. All the fast food and processed snacks have added to our now obese and disease stricken population.

Throughout this chapter we will explore how to use nutrition to your advantage for weight loss and weight maintenance, immune system health, brain power, and anti-aging.

Nutrition and Weight loss

The best way to filter through the multitude of fad diets and quick fixes is to understand how they work (or don't work) and get back to the basic principles of how to get to and maintain a healthy weight. It may come as a surprise to many of our readers, but there is not a fad diet out there that will make you thin and keep you thin. While some may work for a short while, they eventually will all fail. The only way to maintain a healthy size over the course of your life, while maintaining healthy nutrition, is to change your everyday habits.

What Doesn't Work

Over the years, many patients have come to see us bragging about their weight loss, while complaining about a myriad of other issues and side effects. Below is a list of some of the fad diets that we have seen patients try and why they just do not make sense for long term health and weight loss.

The Adkins Diet

This diet was designed as a low-carbohydrate, high fat, high protein diet. The science behind this diet is to make the body burn fat and reduce water at a very fast pace. The body actually takes on a ketogenic state where ketones (broken down fat) are at high levels in the blood stream. This can lead to a dangerous problem called acidosis or ketosis.

A person could actually harm their body in many ways, including reducing the body's T3 cells. In turn, this will decrease your natural ability to metabolize fats and carbohydrates in the future. This diet also causes a loss of water weight due to low carbohydrate intake, which is over compensated once the dieter has stopped the program.

Besides the problems listed above, the excessive intake of fat and protein can increase the potential for heart disease and diabetes. Adkins himself didn't recommend this diet for anyone with kidney problems, diabetes, pregnant or nursing women, etc. While this diet may work for short term weight loss, it is not a viable option for long term health.

Pre-packaged Food Diets

These come in many names and varieties, usually with celebrity paid endorsements about how much weight they have lost. These plans come with pre-packaged food that you have to buy from the supplier, often they must be supplemented with fresh fruits and vegetables that you buy at your local grocery store.

The boxed food is filled with a long list of ingredients including artificial ingredients, preservatives, and synthetic nutrients. This is exactly what we try to keep our patients away from. Not to mention that many of the foods list partially hydrogenated oils (trans-fat). Processed foods combined with low caloric intake causes fatigue and other health issues.

Medifast

This fad diet asks participants to have an average caloric intake of 800-1000 calories per day. It is basically a low fat, low carbohydrate, very low calorie plan that was originally designed to be physician supervised. Like the Adkins diet, this diet works by placing the body in a state of ketosis.

Dieters on this plan are encouraged to drink protein shakes and keep protein levels up. Since Medifast can now be used without physician supervision, dieters are left to monitor themselves. Without proper amounts of protein, muscle and organ damage can occur. Less severe side effects include lightheadedness, confusion, irritability, sleep disturbances, and gastrointestinal problems.

Malnutrition and dehydration are also a concern with any low calorie diet. This, like all diets that work through very low calorie, low carbohydrate, and low fat intake is not a good strategy for long term healthy weight loss.

Diet Drugs

There are many diet drugs, it is impossible to list them all in this chapter. They range from appetite suppressants, to herbal supplements, to fat blockers. Many diet drugs, especially appetite suppressants, have been linked to serious side effects including permanent heart damage.

No diet drugs are designed to be a long term solution to weight loss or weight maintenance. Basically, there is no magical pill.

Now that we have gone through some of the fad diets and explained why they don't work, let's take a look at some lifestyle changes you can make that will help reduce weight and work long term.

The key to long term weight loss is to go back to the basics of healthy nutrition and staying active. Eating healthy is somewhat of a trick these days because labels are misleading, ingredient lists are lengthy, and there are so many options when it comes to food.

Understanding Ingredients

Manufacturers have mastered the art of disguising ingredients so that consumers will buy their products without fully understanding what's really in them. For example, corn syrup, high fructose corn syrup, dextrose, and maltose are all sugar. Ingredients are listed with the most prevalent one being first in the list. Therefore, if any of the terms for sugar are listed first, it means that sugar is the main ingredient.

When reading labels and deciding which foods are best for you, having a clear understanding of how the Food and Drug Administration (FDA) approves labels is helpful. Below is a list of key words that manufacturers use along with what they can legally mean.

Certified Organically Grown: This is the only organic label that matters. All the other terms such as organic, pesticide free, or no artificial ingredients, are often misleading and not monitored.

Lite or *Light*: this can mean that the product has less calories or half the fat of the original version, the item has less sodium, or that it is simply lighter in color.

Low Fat: the item has less than 3 grams of fat per serving. The serving size can be determined as a very small amount of the product, so pay close attention to the "suggested serving size" on the label.

Fat Free: the item has less than .5 grams of fat per serving. Many manufacturers will shrink the serving size to allow the use of this term.

Fortified: the food has been chemically altered in some way

Fruit Drinks: usually means that the drink has been artificially flavored to taste like a fruit flavor. For real fruit, look for labels that read "made with 100% fruit juice"

Natural or *Made from Natural*: this is a term that only means that the manufacturer started with a natural ingredient. The final product can be filled with anything that has been added to that natural source.

Reduced or *Less Fat*: the product contains 25% less fat than their full fat version. So, if a serving size has 12 grams of fat, the reduced fat version may still have 9 grams of fat per serving! (Again, watch the serving size)

Sugar free: this term, along with no sugar added and sugarless, often reflect that the product is filled with artificial sweeteners that are more dangerous than real sugar.

High Fructose Corn Syrup

About ten years ago doctors started seeing an increase in child-hood obesity and many newly diagnosed diabetics. It has become the opinion of many in the medical field that this is caused by the overuse of sugars, especially high fructose corn syrup. New studies also suggest that fructose corn syrup also increases blood pressure in men.

The Institute for Agriculture and Trade policy (IATP) announced in early 2009 that high fructose corn syrup, which is in many of our foods and almost all soft drinks, contains detectable levels of mercury. Mercury is a very dangerous substance even in the smallest amounts. Many medical professionals fear that this finding may have come too late and that the long term effects of mercury exposure may not be known for several years.

Sodium Nitrite (Sodium Nitrate)

This is often found as a preservative in bacon, lunch meat, smoked fish, and hot dogs. Some studies have found a link between Sodium

Nitrite, which converts to nitrosamines, and cancer in humans. It also can cause migraines, so if you are prone to headaches you may want to eliminate this from your diet.

Hydrogenated Vegetable oil or Partially Hydrogenated Vegetable Oil

When this ingredient is listed on the label, trans-fats are present. You will often find this ingredient listed in margarines, cookies, bread, vegetable shortening, sauces and dressings, and much more. Trans-fats have been strongly linked to heart disease and diabetes.

Artificial Food Coloring

With all the natural coloring choices available, it is a shame that manufacturers lean so heavily on artificial food dyes. Many studies have linked these substances to diseases in rats. For example: mice that were exposed to Blue and Blue 2 were more likely to get brain tumors. Likewise, Red 3 caused rats to have a high instance of thyroid tumors. Yellow #6 has been linked to kidney and adrenal tumors in rats as well as asthma in children.

Aspartame

Aspartame is a combination of aspartic acid, phenylalanine, and methanol. Many physicians refer to this as a chemical cocktail. It is found in many diet drinks, gums, sugar free products, and can be packaged as NutraSweet or Equal. In the 1970s there was proof that this product was linked to brain tumors in rats. As recent as 2005, a study linked Aspartame to not just brain tumors, but lymphomas and leukemia in rats.

Many human diseases and disorders can be made worse by the ingestion of this additive. People with Multiple Sclerosis (MS), epilepsy, chronic fatigue syndrome, Parkinson's disease, Alzheimer's, lymphoma, fibromyalgia, and diabetes should avoid all foods with Aspartame.

*The above list is not exhaustive. A good rule of thumb when scanning ingredients is to avoid buying foods that contain a large number of ingredients, especially ones that are hard to pronounce. Sticking to foods that are in their natural state is always best.

The Best Foods for You

There are a number of foods that are loaded with important natural ingredients. These foods, in their natural state, were put on this earth to keep people healthy. By consuming foods filled with natural vitamins and minerals, bodies can look and feel young. Some foods not only have healing properties that boost the immune system, but they also increase brain power and stamina.

When it comes to fruits and vegetables, choose ones that are rich in color. They will contain anthocyanins, which boost the immune system. They will also contain higher levels of vitamins and minerals. Below is a list of fruits and vegetables that you should consume on a regular basis.

Foods That Help You Maintain a Proper Weight

Beans: High in fiber and filled with Cholecystokinin (a natural appetite suppressant) this is a must have in every diet. An added bonus is that beans have also been shown to lower cholesterol.

Cinnamon: One of the most unlikely weight loss secrets of all time. This spice has been shown to curb cravings. A USDA study also showed that it lowered blood sugar and lipid (cholesterol and triglyceride) levels in type II diabetics.

Eggs: Full of protein, eating eggs will help you stay full longer. They have also been shown to prevent spikes in blood sugar that later lead to more food cravings. If you are watching your cholesterol, forgo the yokes and just eat the egg whites.

Grapefruit: Filled with phytochemicals, this fruit actually helps reduce insulin levels, which in turn keeps calories from turning into fat by using them instead for energy. In 2006 a study at the Metabolic Research Center at Scripps Clinic enrolled 91 obese people and found that consuming grapefruit before each meal helped people drop more than three pounds over 12 weeks.

Hot Red Peppers: these contain a natural ingredient, capsaisin, which works as an appetite suppressant. Using them to spice up a meal may keep you from snacking later.

Green Tea: Studies have shown that the catechins in green tea help speed metabolism and reduce body mass index. One Japanese study even showed a drop in LDL (bad cholesterol).

Lean Beef: Surprising, but beef is actually a good component to weight loss. Lean beef is actually filling and plays an important role in protein intake that allows you to lose fat and keep lean muscle mass. Dieters who eat meat also have less hunger pains.

Nuts: Although nuts contain fat, it looks as though the benefits of eating nuts far outweigh their fat calories. A study a Purdue University added nuts to their diet and actually boosted their metabolism by as much as 11%.

Olive Oil: Long known for its health benefits, a study in Australia showed that eating extra virgin olive oil actually boosts metabolism.

Pears: Containing 6 grams of fiber per medium sized pear, they help you feel full and prevent other snacking. The Pectin fiber in pears and apples actually decreases blood sugar levels and fights off cravings. A Brazilian study showed that women who ate 3 pears a day, compared to those that ate 3 oat cookies, lost more weight over a 12 week period.

Salad: Filled with essential vitamins, eating a salad as a start to any meal will make you feel fuller faster and naturally helps you avoid large portions of fat and carbohydrates. Read the labels of dressings and other salad additions in an effort to keep fat and calories to a minimum.

Vinegar: For the people who just can't avoid bread, a Swedish study found that dipping the bread in vinegar may reduce the amount that the person eats. There is also a theory that the acidic acid in vinegar keeps spikes of blood sugar at bay.

Foods That Boost Your Immunity

Avocado: Filled with Vitamin E and C, this vegetable helps rid the body of free radicals. Don't worry about the fat in avocados, studies show that it helps unlock bad fats and excrete them from the system, actually helping maintain weight.

Broccoli: Filled with antioxidants and Vitamins A, C, and E this vegetable should be a regular part of a healthy diet. Broccoli is also high in glucosinolates which boosts the body's immune system and sulforaphanes, which keeps cells from turning cancerous.

Chicken Soup: For years, chicken soup has been the prescription for colds and other illnesses. There is actually science behind why it works so well. Cysteine, an amino acid found in chicken soup is chemically similar to acetylcysteine, a drug used for bronchitis.

The broth works like cough medicine by thinning the mucus.

Fish: High in Omega 3 fatty acids, fish is one of the most powerful immune boosting foods. Two servings a week will help you fight off upper respiratory illness by keeping airways clear.

Garlic: Containing allicin, garlic helps fight off viruses and bacteria. A British study on garlic showed that those who consumed it on a regular basis for 12 weeks were 2/3 less likely to catch a cold. Other studies on garlic have shown it to be affective in fighting off colorectal and stomach cancers.

Ginger: This root will actually help "sweat out" colds and viruses. Not only does it increase the body's ability to sweat, it has anti-inflammatory properties. Ginger is also good for an upset stomach.

Oregano: Herbs and spices are high in antioxidants, but oregano is the highest. Add it to salads, main dishes, anything to fight off colds, flu, infection, and even indigestion.

Pumpkin: Filled with Vitamin A, this vegetable has immune boosting properties that fight off small infections as well as cancer. Since Vitamin A is stored in fat cells, taking it in pill form can increase the risk of toxicity. FDA recommends getting Vitamin A from vegetables such as this one.

Shell Fish: Oysters, lobster, and crab all help the body's white blood cells produce cytokins which fight off the flu virus. Be sure to eat these during flu season, which typically starts in October and ends after January.

Tea: Both black and green teas contain L-theanin, an immune boosting amino acid. A Harvard study showed that people who drank 5 cups of black tea for 14 days had more interferon in their blood. Interferon helps fight viruses. If caffeine is a problem, no worry, decaf tea still contains the amino acid.

Turmeric: Part of traditional Chinese medicine, this spice has cold and flu fighting properties. Use this on chicken and you will get both protein and viral fighting properties. Curcumin, found in turmeric, showed anti-inflammatory properties, in a 2008 study published in Biochemical and Biophysical Research Communications.

Yogurt: Some bacteria are good for the body and essential to proper digestive health. A Swedish study of factory employees showed that those who ingested Lactobacillus Reuteri had 1/3 less sick days over 80 days. Lactobacillus Reuteri is a probiotic that stimulates white blood cells. Not all yogurts have the same probiotics, so check labels.

Foods for a Youthful Appearance

Avocado: The monounsaturated fat (good fat) actually helps boost the plumpness of skin cells giving younger appearance and less visible wrinkles. Studies have also shown that this vegetable helps lower cholesterol, which will keep you young on the inside too.

Beans and lentils: Great for hair and nails. Not only will they grow faster, they will be stronger.

Berries: Eating these will help the body to produce more collagen, a vital protein that keeps skin soft and elastic.

Brazil Nuts: Filled with selenium, eating these nuts will increase the elasticity in hair and skin. High in zinc, they are actually good for the immune system as well.

Buckwheat: Not a grain at all, this fruit of a plant is filled with nutrition, especially amino acids.

Eggs: Full of Vitamin B12, B6, D, and E, along with protein, this food a super food for building lean muscle mass.

Green Tea: Works as an anti-inflammatory agent and reduces the risk of skin cancer.

Salmon: Full of omega-3 fatty acids, this high-quality protein source is also filled with Vitamin B-12 and Iron and will keep your hair and skin healthy and younger looking. It also keeps your scalp from drying out and flaking.

Spinach: This dark green vegetable works as a natural hair conditioner (when eaten, of course).

Water: One of the easiest ways to keep wrinkles and fine lines from being so noticeable is to stay hydrated.

Foods for a Younger Mind

Avocado: This Omega 3 fatty acid packed vegetable is great alone or with a burger. It is proven to give added brain power.

Blueberries: A focus pill in the form of a sweet berry. Blueberries are perfect for those with ADD (Attention Deficit Disorder) and those without.

Dark Chocolate: Tasty and full of antioxidants leaving both the brain and sweet tooth satisfied. The added caffeine also helps with alertness.

Fish: The omega 3 fatty acids found in fish help with mental clarity and fight off dementia.

Kale and *Spinach*: Both these leafy green vegetables have been shown to fight off Alzheimer's disease.

Nuts: With their antioxidant and protein properties, a hand full of these will help you get and stay focused.

Popcorn: Filled with Vitamins B6, B12, and E, this fun food will help boost memory and alertness. The healthiest popcorn is air popped and without butter or salt.

Super Foods

Blueberries: These little berries are packed with a powerful punch of health and wellness. They contain antioxidants and phytoflavinoids and are high in potassium and Vitamin C. They fight off chronic disease and have shown to be helpful in the fight against cancer and heart disease.

Eggs: Forget that eggs are bad for your heart. A study at Harvard proved it to be untrue. Actually, eggs are a super food that fights off macular degeneration, keeps the nervous system healthy, regulates the brain, and decreases the risk of breast cancer. It is one of the few foods that also contains naturally occurring Vitamin D.

Kale: This less popular leafy green vegetable has enormous benefits. Filled with Vitamins and Minerals, it wards off cancers, heart disease, chronic diseases, cataracts, and osteoporosis.

Salmon: Filled with omega 3, this fish has amazing properties. It fights off cancer, boosts brain power, it is good for your heart, lowers blood pressure, regulates mood and is amazing in its ability to steady the roller coaster of bipolar disorder. Little wonder that it takes the title as "One of the Worlds Healthiest Foods!"

Soy: Gaining popularity, soy has many health benefits that are making it a mainstream contender. Benefits include: lowering cholesterol, strengthening bones, and offering relief from menopausal symptoms.

Sweet Potato: Filled with Vitamins A, B1, B6, C, E, potassium, copper, iron, and manganese. They are good for your eyes, skin, hair, brain, teeth, gums, heart, nervous system, and cardiovascular system. They also have anti-inflammatory properties that fight off arthritis, asthma, and allergies. Studies show that sweet potatoes have what it takes to ward off strokes and heart attacks.

Nutrition for Life

Our society has given us almost a limitless number of options when it comes to food. If you are forty years or younger, you may have to separate yourself from the fast food upbringing that you became accustomed to. Getting back to basics is the best way to stay looking and feeling young.

Our recommendations for each day include:

7-9 servings of fruits and vegetables. Best raw or steamed, but never canned. (Make one of these from the list of super foods to get the most benefit.)

6-7 oz. of protein from eggs, beans, meat, or fish (eat fish twice a week.)

2-3 servings of low-fat dairy (unless lactose intolerant)

6-8 servings of whole wheat bread, brown rice, or pasta

64 oz. of water

2-4 cups of tea (black or green)

In an effort to help you track what you are eating, take a moment and fill out the 3 day food diary below.

DAY ONE

BREAKFAST
_____

SNACK
_____

LUNCH
_____

SNACK
_____

DINNER
_____

DAY TWO

BREAKFAST
_____

SNACK
_____

LUNCH
_____

SNACK
_____

DINNER
_____

DAY THREE

BREAKFAST
_____

SNACK
_____

LUNCH
_____

SNACK
_____

DINNER
_____

Take a moment to look at the items recorded above. What things should you have less of? What things should you have more of?

_____

_____

_____

_____

_____

_____

_____

_____

Looking back in through the pages on Nutrition, are there any items that you want to include in your diet to help with your immunity, weight, or libido? List them below and then put them on your grocery list:

_____

_____

_____

_____

_____

_____

_____

_____

Step #4

Go to the Spa

While trips to the spa are not a cure within themselves, it is an important part of health and wellness. It may seem natural to some, while completely unconventional to others, but the idea of using a spa day as a way to regenerate the body and promote good health dates back to 3000 BC. For centuries, massage, reflexology, soaking, and other spa treatments have been used to keep the body in working order and in a state of ease. Even before mankind knew the true dangers of stress, we had found ways to combat it.

Massage Therapy

One of the most popular treatments at any spa is massage. The first writings about massage took place in 2000 BC, and by 776 BC the athletes at the Olympic Games were receiving massages prior to their performance. In 100 AD, the first massage schools began in China. The early world recognized this treatment as a vital part of good health and wellness. However, America was not introduced to the benefits of massage therapy in the mid 1800s.

Today, modern technology has allowed us to measure the benefits of massage. We now know that it increases blood flow, releases endorphins and serotonin, increases the number of T-cells (these cells are important for a healthy immune system), increases the function of the lymphatic system, and elevates overall mood. Massage also puts the body in a state of deep relaxation, which allows the brain to relax and unload stress. In turn, mental functions such as memory and strategic thinking return at a higher level.

Many people view spa treatments as a luxury and not a necessity. This misguided thought is often held in the Western part of the world, and is not necessarily held in other parts. In China, for example, massage and other spa treatments are integrated into primary care and hospital care for patients. In many countries it is not only part of medical treatment, but sometimes even covered by the government sponsored health program.

In the United States, recent research is gaining the attention of mainstream medicine, including some listed in the Archives of Internal Medicine. A study that was published in the Archives showed promising results for patients with osteoarthritis. The University of Medicine and Dentistry of New Jersey and the Yale Prevention Research Center conducted the study which incorporated massage therapy into half of the research subjects in a study on osteoarthritis of the knee. After eight weeks, the group that had massages added to their medical regimen showed increased mobility and decreased pain. These results remained consistent even after an additional eight weeks off of treatment. They later received a $1.4 Million grant from the federal government for a study to determine the optimal dosing regimen of massage in osteoarthritis treatment.

Studies, such as the one above, have become popular among medical schools and university hospitals. The results are overwhelmingly in favor of massage as a way to help treat illness as well as promote overall health. On the following page is a list of just some of the benefits of massage as proven through research studies:

- Mothers who are mourning over the loss of a child are less likely to suffer severe depression

- Students can reduce stress and anxiety before an exam

- Athletes are more likely to perform at peak levels

- The immune system of both ill and well patients are boosted due to increased white cells and T-cells

- HIV exposed infants have increased weight gain and are more likely to thrive

- Premature babies had increased weight gain

- Patients who undergo abdominal surgery are likely to heal faster

- Patients experience decreased blood pressure

- Migraine sufferers see a decrease in number and intensity

- Office workers increase alertness and performance levels

- Weak and inactive muscles are stimulated, partially compensating for their lack of activity

- Muscles relax and range of motion is increased

- Patients who suffer from anxiety or depression have a decrease in symptoms

- Lower back pain sufferers often find long term relief after several treatments

- Autistic children showed a decrease in erratic behavior

- Stroke patients showed a significant increase in quality of life, used less medication, and had better mobility

- Cancer patients had less pain and anxiety

- Burn patients experienced less pain, itching, and irritability

- After treatment, patients showed an increase in brain alertness evidenced by EEG patterns. Mathematical computation was also faster and more accurate

- Decreased symptoms in subclinical depression

While there are multiple studies that could fill many pages of this book, the above list is just a snapshot of what the modern world is beginning to understand about the benefits of massage and is supported by the power of respected clinical studies.

Reflexology

Reflexology was created by the Egyptians in 2500 BC. Today, it is a part of many chiropractic and osteopathic practices. It was introduced in America in 1913 by an ear, nose and throat doctor by the name of William H. Fitzgerald. It was later further developed by a nurse and physiotherapist named Eunice Ingham, who is closely linked to the form of reflexology practiced in the United States today.

Although there is benefit in reflexology, it must be made clear that we do not suggest this or any other spa treatment as a sole treatment for any disease or disorder. There is much controversy in the medical community surrounding the delay of treatment for disease in patients who seek alternative treatments as sole treatments for their condition. That said, understanding the role that reflexology plays in the health and wellness of the body can provide great benefit, granted it is not offered as a front line or sole treatment method.

This treatment involves massaging or applying controlled pressure to parts of the feet, hands, and ears. The purpose is to promote health in other parts of the body that are believed to be linked or connected in some way. Much like the name suggests, pressure in one area would offer relief in another area of the body.

One of the biggest problems with the use of reflexology as a part of modern medical care is its lack of controlled clinical trials that study its effect. Many respected medical journals and medical institutions have reviewed previous studies for their legitimacy and have found that their positive results were not gathered in a fashion that would hold up to recognized research standards. The studies that are being done and currently hold legitimacy are in the areas of multiple sclerosis and pain treatment.

Many studies have been conducted using reflexology in the treatment of premenstrual syndrome, circulatory related diseases, and hormonal deficiencies. While there may be some benefit, in our medical judgment, it should only be used in addition to modern treatments and never in place of them. Reflexology does have its place in the world of health and wellness. How it may benefit a particular patient is based on many factors and continuation of such treatment is at the discretion of each patient. We have had several patients who have benefited by its use for relief from stress or headaches, while others did not see any.

We do know, however, that the principles of reflexology have been proven through the use of medical technology. With the use of a functional MRI (fMRI) doctors have been able to physically see the brain reacting to pressure points. The reactions within the brain do show a relationship between the points and the expected corresponding body part as described by modern reflexology text books. More study is needed to understand how the relationship relates to treatment of different conditions.

Safety and Spa Use

In the United States, only 37 states regulate massage therapists. While massage is a beneficial form of treatment for many, it can be dangerous if not performed by a licensed and experience massage therapist. Always check the spa that you will be attending to be sure that they have verified the licenses of the therapists that work for them.

When having a massage, be sure that your therapist is listening to you. A massage should never be painful and you must communicate to ensure that the pressure is safe for your body. Beware of a pushy therapist and if you are feeling rough-handled, ask them to discontinue the massage.

As a customer, it is your job to inform the spa of any allergies or sensitivities that you may have to oils, foods, or perfumes. Some oils may contain ingredients that are not best for sensitive skin. Be sure to communicate any of these concerns with your therapist before your treatment. If at any time during your treatment you feel itching or burning, be sure to let them know.

Many spas have saunas and steam rooms. If you are pregnant it is not safe to use these facilities. You should also avoid these if you have any serious medical conditions, including high or low blood pressure, heart disease, asthma or epilepsy. If you are healthy and do partake in the sauna and/or steam room, be sure to use shoes and a towel. Direct contact with the surfaces will put you at increased risk for skin infections like fungus.

Using good judgment and keeping in constant communication with those who will be servicing you will make your visit not only more enjoyable but much safer too. Incorporating spa treatments into your routine can have many health benefits when done right.

The Power of Touch

Touch is the first sense we receive, usually developing as early as eight weeks, and the last sense to leave us as we die. In today's touch free society, we are seeing an increase in stress and depression. While a day at the spa may be in order to get a dose of touch therapy, simple changes in habits could be beneficial. Remember to hug your kids and spouse. Don't be afraid to give a pat on the back (or receive one).

In response to the concern over the lack of touch; touch is being scientifically studied as it relates to medicine and health. The Touch Research Institute was developed by Tiffany Field, Ph.D., of the University of Miami School of Medicine.   It was established with the use of a grant from Johnson & Johnson. The study of touch is also gaining attention from researchers from Harvard, Duke, Maryland and other well respected universities.

In one study, a neuroscientist at the University of Virginia found that women who were under stress found immediate relief through the touch of their spouses hand. Through the use of a functional MRI scan, women were exposed to a mild shock, but when their spouse held their hand, there was a decrease in brain response, showing that the patient was less stressed. While the effect was less, they also saw relief with the touch of a stranger.

Studies have long shown the benefits of touch in infants, as well as the devastating effects the lack of touch can have. Many years ago, the media covered the story of Romanian Orphanages. They exposed the devastating effects of not being touched. The babies had been fed and clothed, but there were not enough workers to hold and rock them. The lack of touch resulted in a failure to thrive and the babies did not grow or develop normally.

Humans need touch to grow and develop. There are over 5 million touch receptors, with over 3,000 in the tip of a finger. These receptors act like signals for the release of endorphins, chemicals within the body that make you feel pleasure and promote happiness. It has been said that touch is as much of a necessity as food and shelter and that the current population, especially in America, is suffering from touch deprivation.

The power of touch has shown to be important in every stage of life. Clinical studies have shown that the same principles of touch, as they apply to infants, have correlated with the ability to thrive with the elderly. There has also been evidence that health and wellness both physically and mentally is dependent on touch at every age and stage of life.

Touch, even when it is not consciously experienced, has a positive effect on the brain. In a study of patrons at a library, a group of participants were lightly touched by the librarian, in a fashion that was not obvious, while the other participants entered and left the library without any form of touch. The group that was "accidentally" touched reported a better experience at the library. Another study which involved dining in a restaurant found that those who were touched by the waitress found the food to be better, reported a positive eating experience, and tipped at higher percentages.

The power of touch is much stronger than most people understand. With the use of functional MRI and other modern methods of study, we will find that touch is not only an important part of relationships, but a vital part of daily health and wellness.

As part of this step to Ultimate Health, take the time to become more aware of your habits as they pertain to this chapter. Take time to answer the questions below. This will help you get a better understanding of how you can apply the principles taught in this step.

On a scale of 1-10 (ten being highest) what stress level do I generally run at?_____

Take one week and log the amount and type of down time that you have provided yourself with:

MONDAY　_____

TUESDAY　_____

WEDNESDAY　_____

THURSDAY　_____

FRIDAY　_____

Saturday　_____

Sunday　_____

Take out your calendar and schedule an appointment with yourself for *"me"* time. Preferably make this a time of relaxation at a spa or a place where you can receive massage therapy.

Think about and make notes that describe your feelings about touch. Do you come from a touchy family or one that was more stand-offish? How has this affected your ability to accept and deliver positive touch with others?

_____

_____

_____

_____

_____

Keep a log for one week of how often you were touched by another or reached out to touch someone else. Also note your overall mood of the day (happy, sad, stressed, etc.)

DAY	NUMBER OF TOUCHES	OVERALL MOOD
MONDAY		
TUESDAY		
WEDNESDAY		
THURSDAY		
FRIDAY		
Saturday		
Sunday		

The purpose of this exercise is to help you recognize touch deprivation and take steps to incorporate touch into your daily activities, especially with family.

Step #5

Adopt an Exercise Program

The health benefits of exercise come as no surprise. Exercise is an important part of daily activity that is necessary to maintaining a healthy weight, a high energy level, mental health, and good blood chemistry. For generations, it wasn't necessary to join a gym or schedule time for a workout because daily living involved a great amount of physical exertion just to survive. Today, very few people live off the land or have jobs that involve aerobic exercise.

A change in the workforce, from physical labor to more sedentary positions, has taken a toll on the health and wellness of the general population. We have seen an increase in the number of people who suffer depression, diabetes, obesity, and a number of related conditions. Taking exercise out of our way of life has changed not only the shape of people today, but has increased their risk for a multitude of diseases and disorders.

Research shows that people who remain active live longer and have a much lower risk of developing or dying from high blood pressure, heart disease, diabetes, and colon cancer. To increase longevity, you must remain active by participating in some sort of physical activity at least once a week. Developing a regular pattern of exercise (2-5 times a week) is best. Most people make the mistake of thinking that there is only benefit in high intensity workouts that leave you covered in sweat and sore for days. The truth is, simple activities such as going for a walk several times a week will yield health benefits.

In 2007 researchers at the Fred Hutchison Cancer Center in Seattle conducted one of the largest studies on the health benefits of exercise. They enrolled 202 healthy men and women ages 40-75 who reported having a sedentary lifestyle. They divided them into two groups; one was a control group where they maintained their current lifestyle, while the others were involved in an exercise program. The exercise group participated in moderate to vigorous exercise for one hour, six days a week.

During the study, female exercisers lost an average of 5.5 percent of intra-abdominal fat, while men lost 7.5 percent over the course of one year. Intra-abdominal fat, which can be measured by CT or MRI, is related to a number of diseases, including cancer, heart disease, and diabetes. This type of fat, also referred to as visceral fat, is often hidden because it is deposited around the internal organs and within the abdominal cavity. Through exercise, visceral fat can be significantly reduced.

Exercise for Heart Health

Giving the heart a good work out can increase your cardiovascular health by lowering blood pressure and positively affecting lipid levels within the blood. High blood pressure can lead to heart attacks, strokes, and kidney disease. An ideal resting blood pressure is less than 115/75 mmHg. A regular exercise routine can help reduce systolic (top number) blood pressure. A brisk walk, cycling or even swimming can positively affect blood pressure when done on a regular basis. According to the US Department of Health and Human Services, maintaining a normal body weight (see the BMI chart on page 73) can reduce systolic pressure as much as 20 mmHg.

Lipid levels, mostly referred to as cholesterol and triglycerides, are also positively influenced by exercise. A study conducted by the University of North Carolina at Chapel Hill studied more than 15,000 men and women for more than twenty years. The study found that exercise increased HDL (good cholesterol) levels and decreased triglyceride levels.

Another study that was published in the American Journal of Medicine found that cardiovascular exercise is associated with a 50% reduction in cardiovascular disease in men. The study also showed that an increase in physical activity in men also gave them a 20% lower mortality rate, thus increasing their life span. The New England Journal of Medicine also published a study in 2004 showing that leading a sedentary lifestyle can double the mortality rate in women.

Exercise for Mental Wellness

When we exercise, our brains release serotonin, a chemical that regulates mood. Many times when people get upset or stressed they go for a walk and calm down. It works because the body is preprogrammed to calm itself down and regulate bad feelings. A number of studies have found that exercise is a major factor in reducing stress, anxiety, and depression.

A study conducted at Duke University found that exercise can be just as effective as anti-depressants in controlling major depressive disorder. In a study of 156 patients with diagnosed depression, they found little difference in the effectiveness of exercise only, exercise and medication, and medication only groups. Maybe one of the most significant findings of this study is that people can be treated naturally for depression without being subject to the side effects of antidepressant medications.

In 2007 the American Journal of Epidemiology published a study about the effects of exercise on anxiety. The University of Bristol followed 1,158 middle-aged British men for ten years. They found that those men who got regular vigorous exercise were less likely to develop anxiety or depression over time. This study is consistent with a number of other studies showing a link between exercise and a lower risk for depressive disorders.

Exercise for Brain Health

According to Brian Christie, a Neuroscientist at the University of Victoria, exercise can actually increase your brain size and make you smarter. During exercise, acetycholine, a neurotransmitter is activated, our level of neutrophins increase, and brain cells are produced. The brains of people that take up walking three times a week have an increase in brain size in as short as three months.

Exercise can help reduce the risk of Alzheimer's disease and dementia. New studies show that thirty minutes of moderate exercise, five times a week, can reduce your risk for Alzheimer's by thirty five percent. Even more impressive is that those that add weight and strengthening exercises to their aerobic workout can cut their risk in half. During Alzheimer's and dementia progression, the brain actually shrinks, but exercise can counteract that process.

Other studies have shown that patients that do develop Alzheimer's have a slower rate of progression if they have had a life of physical activity. Those that have lived a more sedentary lifestyle in the past tend to deteriorate at a much faster rate.

Exercise for Weight Loss

Exercising on a regular basis will help the body maintain a healthy weight. There are a number of benefits to weight loss that include lower risk for diseases such as diabetes, less strain on the joints, a healthier heart, and a better self-esteem. In 1999 the US reported that 61% of its population was overweight. This number has increased drastically from 1970 and continues to climb.

Exercise plays a significant role in reducing weight. Diet alone, is not the answer to weight loss, because long term weight loss is dependent on lean muscle mass. Making physical activity part of your daily routine will help you live longer and healthier. If you have children, it is especially important to make exercise part of the routine for the family. Doing so will prevent generational obesity problems, and help everyone in the family have a better overall quality of life.

Exercise to Help Arthritis

While vigorous exercise may be contraindicated for advanced arthritis, low-impact to moderate levels of exercise has shown great benefit. Water aerobics is a great way for those with arthritis to enjoy the benefits of exercise without damaging already fragile joints. A recent study showed that participants that took part in a community based water aerobics program showed less arthritic pain and a higher mobility rate. They also had an increased range of motion in the hips, allowing them to go up and down stairs easier and without as much pain.

The University of North Carolina at Chapel Hill studied 346 adults in an effort to see if the arthritic participants would react favorably to exercise. The participants were put through the PACE (People with Arthritis Can Exercise) program that was developed by The Arthritis Foundation. At the conclusion of the study, the researchers found that participants have general improvement in both pain and fatigue.

If you suffer from arthritis or fibromyalgia, it is a good idea to find a low impact exercise program, like water aerobics, to participate in. Living a sedentary lifestyle will only make the symptoms and conditions worse. Take time to visit with your doctor to decide what exercise program is best for your condition.

Exercise to Prevent Diabetes

The lack of exercise has devastating effects on the body's insulin regulatory mechanisms. Type 2 diabetes is a very dangerous condition that is related to multiple complications, including early death. Exercise is a natural way to prevent diabetes, and decrease the effects of the disease for those who already have it. New research shows that regular exercise is the number one factor in preventing, and controlling diabetes.

In 2001 a study conducted at Brown University found that diet and exercise can decrease the chance of developing diabetes in those at high risk. Following a proper diet and adding exercise can decrease the risk by 58 percent. The study included 3,234 people and was conducted at 27 medical centers throughout the United States. Simply taking a brisk walk or doing other physical activity for thirty minutes a day would reduce the risk of diabetes and lessen the number of people afflicted by the disease, which is now exceeds 16 million.

While any exercise should be under the supervision of your physician, the most effective fitness program for diabetes prevention involves aerobic, resistance, and flexibility training. This combination gives the best results in reducing body fat and increasing lean muscle mass.

Exercise to Reduce Menopausal Symptoms

Menopause often comes with a plethora of less than enjoyable side effects, from mood swings, hot flashes, and headaches, to loss of bone mass. A number of new studies show that exercise can benefit women who are in this stage of their life. The University of Erlangen in Germany found that women who participate in a regular exercise program had increased bone density, fewer mood swings, less headaches and were able to sleep better.

Women tend to gain a significant amount of weight during and after menopause. New studies done in the United States and Australia have found that the weight gain is not due to diet changes, but instead is caused by a drastic reduction in physical activity. If women increase activity, or at the very least keep the same amount of activity as they had ten years earlier, they would not see such a change in their weight.

Exercise to Fight Cancer

Our body has natural defenses that help it stay healthy. Sometimes those defenses can be down due to stress or inactivity. Exercise and physical activity are actually very important to our body's natural defense mechanisms. When we exercise we may be more successful in fighting off cancer and other diseases.

New research shows that there may be significant link to exercise and two types of cancer: colon and breast. The University of California studied 3,000 men with colon cancer and compared them to the general male population of Los Angeles County. The men that had jobs requiring them to be less active had a 60% higher risk of colon cancer.

Women who exercise were found to have a significantly lower risk of breast cancer. This may be due to a later start time of their menstrual cycle and lower body fat, nonetheless, it is an important finding. A review of 25,000 death records showed that those women with a sedentary job had a higher risk for developing breast cancer while those with more demanding jobs and those who were athletes had a much lower risk.

Some researchers argue that exercise reduces all cancer risks because it lowers stress levels. Chemicals released during exercise keep negative feelings at bay. In turn, the body is able to fight off diseases, such as cancer, much easier. Exercise also produces other chemicals that produce more healthy cells and reduce the number of mutations.

Exercise for Better Sex

The irony is that sex is exercise, but exercise outside of sex increases the desire for more intercourse, while increasing the quality of such relations. Exercise seems to "prime" both the male and female for more satisfying sexual activity.

Good circulation is critical to a healthy erection. Doctors at the New England Research Institute found that men who incorporate vigorous exercise into their weekly routines have a lower risk of impotence. The University of California, San Diego found that men who began an exercise program had more satisfying and more frequent sex.

The benefits of exercise and sex are not limited to just men. A study at the University of Texas found that women who exercised vigorously for 20 minutes had an increased blood flow to the genitals and a 169% greater vaginal response to sexually stimulated images.

Best Time to Exercise

As physicians we are often asked when the best time is to exercise. The answer depends on the reason for exercise. For example, if exercise is mostly for mental clarity and energy, an early morning walk is best. However, if the goal is to lose weight, it is best to save your exercise routine until the late afternoon.

Our bodies are set to a circadian clock and our body temperature fluctuates throughout the day. If you are really serious about burning calories, the American Council on Exercise suggests that you take your temperature every two hours (during waking hours of course) for three days. Because body temperature varies throughout the day, your readings may be plus or minus 1.5 degrees. You should be able to determine the time of day that you are at your circadian peak by finding when you have your highest temperature. The best time to exercise, for the purpose of weight loss, is when your temperature is the highest, thus allowing more calories to be burned.

Any time of the day that you can exercise is a good time. It is better to get some exercise in then to avoid it because it wasn't the "right" time of day. If you are training for an athletic event, such as a run or triathlon, it is best to train at the same time of day as the event that you will be participating in. Your body will program itself to be at top performance during that time, making you more effective at the time of the event.

Important Components of an Effective Exercise Program

While encouraging each person to do something to increase their activity level, we want to point out the components that an effective exercise program should involve. In your efforts to maximize the benefits available, try to engage in a program that has the following:

Aerobic Exercise: Also referred to as "cardio", this is the type of exercise that gets your heart rate up. It usually involves something like running, jumping rope, or dancing. In order to achieve aerobic level exercise your heart rate should be between 60-80% of your maximal heart rate. A general guide is to take 220 and subtract your age to get your maximal heart rate. Your pulse (heart beats per minute) should fall between 60-80% of that number.

Strengthening Exercises: This type of exercise is accomplished with resistance or weight lifting. The goal is to work all the major muscle groups, so your arms, chest, back, abdomen, and legs should each be engaged.

Flexibility Exercises: Often referred to as "stretching", these are low-impact and offer great benefits. You should use stretching exercises as a way to warm-up and cool-down in conjunction with the rest of your exercise.

In Conclusion

The main point of this step is to get moving and to enjoy the many health benefits that exercise and physical activity have to offer. We want to encourage you to get moving and improve your level of involvement in your health. Be patient and be consistent, you will see results. Below are a few simple steps that you can take to increase your mobility:

- Chose a parking spot that is far from the entry to the store. This is a great way to add a few steps to your day.

- When you have the choice, take the stairs and skip the elevator.

- Take 5 minute breaks at work and stretch. This will help increase blood flow and stimulate tired muscles.

- Pick either the morning or evening, but walk your block at least 3 days a week.

- When your car is dirty, wash it by hand. This is a great way to incorporate all the components of a good work out into a 30-45 minute session.

- Do 20 jumping jacks a day for a week, then add 10 more each week until you reach 100 per day. (Hint: doing these naked in front of a mirror will encourage you to do more exercise!)

- Have sex (with all precautions of course) 3 times a week. Consider it "exercise with benefits".

Below is a way to help you identify your exercise habits. Answer the questions honestly to get the most benefit:

On average, how often do I exercise each week?

- ☐ I don't exercise on a regular basis
- ☐ I try to exercise at least 3 times a week
- ☐ I exercise almost every day
- ☐ I exercise more than once a day

What were my exercise habits as a child?

☐ I was an active child that participated in sports

☐ I played outside and got plenty of activity

☐ I usually had a moderate amount of exercise, but nothing routine

☐ I was a couch potato

List 3 ways that you can improve your activity level

_____

_____

_____

List the 3 top reasons why you need to improve in this area (example: heart health, mental benefits, etc.)

_____

_____

_____

NOW IS THE TIME TO TAKE ACTION AND TAKE CONTROL OF YOUR HEALTH.
GOOD LUCK IN YOUR EFFORTS TO BECOME MORE ACTIVE AND STAY YOUNG.

Step #6

Get Spiritually Centered

The World Health Organization (WHO) defines true health as "a state of complete physical, mental, and social well-being." This is significant because leaders from around the world recognize that health and wellness transcend the physical health and lack of disease. It encompasses a balance with the human mind, body, and spirit. The Western world is probably the last to fully appreciate the connection, while ancient societies have long understood the concept.

The current political structure in America emphasizes a separation of church and state, but new research shows that there is a link between spiritual health and physical health. Albert Einstein stated, "Science without religion is lame. Religion without science is blind." What seems to have happened is a bidding war over particular religions, rather than an appreciation for the human spirit's need for a higher power, regardless of how that need is expressed. However, new research, including some that is funded through the National Institute of Health (NIH), is showing a positive connection between spiritual and physical health.

Studies have shown that patients who participate in religion, regardless of denomination, have a lower occurrence of heart disease and stroke. Some research shows that the belief system of a higher power is also connected with less anxiety, depression, and stress; naturally followed by a lower suicide rate. Those attending religious ceremonies (church, synagogue, etc.) also have a lower rate of alcoholism and drug abuse. The relationship between spiritual health and physical health is becoming overwhelmingly obvious.

A recent review published on WebMD looked at the medical literature on religion and mortality. The review showed 42 studies that involved a total of 126,000 people and revealed that those who participated in religious activities were more likely to live longer. During the different studies, those who were practicing their religious beliefs were also 29% more likely to be alive at the end of the study than those with no religious affiliation.

There are a number of reasons that scientists use to explain why those that spend time increasing their spiritual health tend to have longer and happier lives. One belief is that the level of stress is reduced when a person has a network of individuals to turn to in times of turmoil. Another is that the very beliefs of most religions revolve around taking care of the body and living a healthier lifestyle. Lastly, the act of meditation or prayer actually changes the physiological and biological factors of one's body and mind.

All of the above are founded on sound reasoning. We know the terrible effects that stress can have on the body. Everything from heart disease, depression, cancer, and many other diseases have been associated with stress either causing the disease or potentially making it worse. Having a social safety net of people with similar beliefs helps alleviate some of the pressures of life. Also, believing in a higher power takes unnecessary stress off people, allowing them to relax and lessen the need to control everything. There is no stress greater than someone trying to control every aspect of their universe, a task that is a lesson in futility.

Religions, regardless of denomination, generally are based around basic principles that are healthy. The fact that they frown on things like alcohol and drug use, makes the believers less likely to partake in those behaviors, or at the very least limit them. Taking care of the human body and spirit is at the center of most beliefs and the social pressure from others within the same belief system may also keep people from harming themselves and associating with those who do.

Most religions involve some sort of prayer or meditation aspect. New studies use modern medical technology to actually show the brain before and after prayer. Andrew Newberg, a neuroscientist at The University of Pennsylvania, has scanned brains for over ten years. Using all types of affiliations, including Tibetan Buddhists and Franciscan nuns, he has gathered information that proves the link between spiritual health and wellbeing. Brain scans confirm that there is an increase in blood flow to particular parts of the brain, along with a decrease to other parts. The brain can shut down the part that takes in sensory information from the outside, and focus on the inside.

Richard Davidson, a neuroscientist at the University of Wisconsin believes that the brain can be sculpted and changed much like the muscles. Science shows that the use of prayer or mediation can actually increase attention and compassion, lessoning communication breakdowns and reducing temper flares. By regularly changing the brain's activity, as evidenced by brain scans, the body begins to recognize and adapt to new neuropathways, a term now coined "neuroplasticity." Davidson claims that not only can the brain change, but recent studies show that the immune system can be boosted as well when one meditates or prays. It appears that spiritual health is a way to self preservation.

During prayer or meditation, the left prefrontal cortex of the brain is activated. This portion of the brain is responsible for positive thoughts like happiness and also controls emotions. A study completed by Davidson, showed that activity in this area was stronger and quicker to activate in a trained mind (like a monk), than in an untrained mind (someone who doesn't participate regularly in prayer or meditation). This new research shows how the brain can be "rewired" to think and act in a more positive manner, but that it takes repetitive action to make those changes.

The benefits of meditation and prayer are overwhelming and the research has just begun to unfold. So many times we see patients who do better than expected when they make their spiritual health as important as their physical health. We are often asked how to get started in the process finding peace in the spirit and mind. While we are doctors, not religious leaders, below are a few tips on meditative prayer.

Start by reading an inspirational passage. This may be from the Bible or other religious book. If religion is not for you, try an inspirational reading from another source.

Create a dark or dimly lit room that is without distraction.

Turn off phones, radios, televisions, and other objects that make noise.

Sit in a still position. It is usually best to sit cross legged on the floor, but if flexibility is a problem you can adapt to whatever is comfortable.

Begin thinking about what you read. Meditate on the words and meanings behind the reading.

To begin or lengthen your meditative state, repeat the Lord's Prayer or other religious prayer several times. The repetition will help block out thoughts about outside issues.

Meditation is most beneficial when done on a regular basis and for long enough to allow the brain function to change. Try to meditate for 20-30 minutes per day to get the best benefit. Schedule meditational prayer just like you would any other appointment. This is an appointment with yourself and should not be seen as a disposable option should a better offer for your time come up. Look for changes in mood and concentration levels as you journey on to a healthier spirit.

Make some notes below that will help you in your journey.

What is the best time for me to schedule meditational prayer?

_____

_____

_____

_____

_____

Where is the best place in my house to practice my meditation?

_____

_____

_____

_____

_____

Am I active in my church, synagogue, or other religiously affiliated community?

_____

_____

_____

_____

_____

If not, list a few places that you like to visit and try to find one that is comfortable:

_____

_____

_____

_____

_____

Keep a journal of your spiritual journey. Make notes about how you are improving your Spiritual life. This will help you stay on task. Keeping in by your bedside and journaling before going to sleep, or when you awaken is best because there are less distractions and allows you a few minutes to think about your journal entry.

Step #7

Take Control of Your Work and Home Life

There are so many factors that make up our personal environment. In a single day we may be at the office, in another state or country, and at home. Each one of these places present completely different environmental factors each with their own health implications.

Taking time to assess your environment will make you more sensitive to how it affects your health. For example, high stress can lead to a multitude of health problems. Finding ways to reduce stress will help you live longer and stay younger and healthier.

A Healthy Home Environment

As physicians we see so many people that suffer from less than satisfactory home lives. A number of issues may contribute to the dissatisfaction, but they usually have something to do with finances, attitude, or a communication breakdown. Even though the issues may be very complex, they inevitably come back to one of these core problems.

Finances: Money is not the answer to happiness, but trouble with finances can lead to an unhappy situation quickly. Research has shown consistently that finances are the number one stressor in personal life and relationships. Worrying about finances can lead to headaches, stomach aches, and insomnia. Arguing about finances can lead to divorce, which comes with its own set of health issues.

Knowing your personal financial situation is the best way to overcome the stress of debt. To most people this seems counterintuitive, but creating a budget and devising a plan to get out of debt is good for your health. Our brains are able to calm down with the "known" but ramp up and misfire with the "unknown".

Debt can actually cause heart disease, obesity, and has been linked to diabetes. When a person has financial stress, their body reacts by releasing adrenaline and cortisol every time they think about it. This increases the heart rate, blood pressure and causes the muscles to tense up. The body also responds to mental stress by dumping glucose and fats into the blood stream.

Taking proactive steps to understand and to improve your financial situation will actually help you live longer. Devise a system that will allow you to turn things around and reduce the strain it is putting on your health. If finances aren't your thing, ask around for a referral to a financial advisor. When you take charge of your finances you will see your health and relationships improve. Several church groups and book clubs run programs based on the book *Financial Peace University* by Dave Ramsey. We highly recommend it and urge you to go through the program.

Attitude: You may have heard it said that "attitude is everything". There is much truth to that statement, especially when dealing with your home life. Stress in the home is often due to the attitude of those that live there. Just like the flu, attitude is contagious. If one person in the home enters the room with a bad attitude it can infect everyone, and change the social climate almost immediately.

Not only is it unpleasant to be around those with a bad attitude, having one yourself can have significant health consequences. The

Mayo Clinic studied 800 people for 30 years and found that those who had a bad attitude were 20 percent more likely to die early than those who were optimists. Therefore, keeping a positive attitude can add years to your life.

The brain is a powerful tool and often our thoughts can actually lead to a self fulfilling prophecy. The more you speak negatively and talk about things that could happen, the more likely they are to come to pass. You are actually training your brain to make subconscious decisions that will favor that outcome. This has been studied and proven over and over. One of the most interesting studies on the topic appeared in the Journal of Psychological Science and looked at people and their attitude on aging. Yale University and the National Institute on Aging looked at 386 men and women and how they viewed older people. They began the study in 1968 and after nearly four decades, those that thought of getting older as a negative thing filled with health issues were significantly more likely to have heart attacks and strokes than those that viewed aging in a positive light.

An earlier study found that those who had a positive attitude about aging eventually lived on average 7.5 years longer than those with negative attitudes. Some researchers believe that the brain can actually sabotage the future if you let a bad attitude take root. This is true in all aspects of attitude, not just in the aspects of aging.

Keeping a positive attitude will increase your level of happiness and deepen your relationships. A positive attitude is just as contagious as a negative one, so go out and infect those around you with good vibes!

Good Communication: One of the greatest lines of any movie came from *Cool Hand Luke*. The infamous "What we have here is a failure to communicate" is so classic that it could be the motto for almost all conflict in life. Communication is a very important aspect of a happy home life and personal tranquility.

The best way to improve communication is to become a good listener. If you are listening, you are not thinking of what you want to say next. Try to become fully engaged in conversations with those around you. Listening to what people have to say and understanding their needs will strengthen personal and professional relationships and improve your health.

Just as you need to be a good listener, you also need to communicate your needs and expectations. This may not come easy and may require practice. If you think people can read your mind and expect them to know what you want, unfortunately you will be let down time and time again. If communicating is hard for you, try first writing things down so that you can organize your thoughts. Then present what you have to say in a non-threatening and informative way. Being a good communicator helps reduce stress because it allows you to get out thoughts instead of leaving them to race through your head.

A Healthy Work Environment

The average American spends more quality waking hours at work than they do at home. Having a healthy work environment is a large part of living a healthy life and maintaining overall wellness. While work conditions have improved from decades ago, and people are not subject to as many hazardous materials as they once were, there are new concerns. Doctors know first-hand that there are health hazards that are seen and unseen, and some cause immediate dangers while others take years to surface. Mental stress and physical stress can take years off of your life. It has been said that Americans now get paid more to live less. There is a dark truth to that statement that echoes in the hearts and minds of all those that have become slave to the 60-hour workweek, Blackberries, and extensive business traveling.

Stress

Stress at work can cause a number of health issues. A study conducted in 1998 looked at the stress levels of 46,000 employees and found that those with high stress at work had 50% more health care costs. Of course, more health care costs are directly associated with more illness.

Work place stress can often be self induced. Some of the best advise we can give patients is not to suffer from MSU (make stuff up). While this is not a diagnosis that you can find in any medical text book, it can create a great deal of unnecessary stress. Basically it works like this: Sally enters a room and finds that the two people within that room become quiet and stop talking. She assumes that they must have been talking about her. She obsesses all day over what they must have said. Later she goes to bring a piece of paper to her boss and finds her boss to be a little short with her. Sally goes home that night and convinces herself that she is being fired and the two other people must already know.

The truth is that the two people that stopped talking were actually in a conversation about one of their children that is having problems. One person was confiding in the other. They got quiet because they didn't want to make the topic common knowledge. Sally's boss had just hung up the phone with her husband after a heated debate prior to Sally dropping off the paper. Neither of these circumstances had anything to do with Sally, yet she has a serious case of MSU and suffered high amounts of stress over it. Long term MSU can lead to high blood pressure, heart disease, obesity, and a number of other health problems.

If you suffer from MSU, here is the only way to cure (or at least control) it:

Calm down and remember that everything isn't always about you.

When you recall the situation, put it through the test: Do I know this is fact? Did I actually hear or see that, or is it MSU?

Think about the overall impact of the situation (facts only). Even if what you experienced is factual, how much does it matter?

Stress at work never stays at the office, it follows the worker home. Tension within the workplace increases tension within the home. The opposite is also true and a study at the Kansas State University showed that employees who found their jobs fulfilling also had happier home lives. So finding and keeping a fulfilling job could actually save a marriage.

Safe at Work

No matter where you work, your work space should be comfortable and safe. Many workplace injuries are completely avoidable. Below are a few tips for staying healthy within your work space:

- Keep the computer screen at an arm's length away

- Tilt the computer screen up 5-15% to reduce glare and prevent headaches

- Use a comfortable chair with lumbar support

- When typing, arms should be in line with hands to avoid carpal tunnel syndrome

- If you work outside, in construction, or in healthcare – follow all OSHA guidelines carefully to limit exposure to hazardous situations

- If you work outside, use sunscreen (SPF 30) to avoid premature aging and skin cancer

- Always go to work well rested – sleepiness accounts for many work injuries

Take time to learn the rules and regulations on safety and understand the health hazards that your particular job posses. Being proactive about your safety at work may just save your life.

Find Balance

In today's fast paced world, it is often hard to find a good balance in how to spend our time. There always seems to be one side that is more demanding than the other. Research shows that people who spend too much time at work have a higher risk for conflict at home.

Workaholism is a serious illness and should be treated as one. Workaholics, like alcoholics, use work as an excuse to escape from other stressors. Although we often think that burying ourselves in work will help make things better, it only makes the situation worse. Furthermore, workaholics have higher levels of heart disease, depression, and strokes.

Workaholics were once praised for their commitment to the job, but the trend is shifting and more companies understand the illness and its implications not only on the person, but the company as a whole. If you suffer from workaholism, talk to your doctor about it.

There is a wonderful book by Bryan E. Robinson, PhD entitled *Chained to the Desk: A Guidebook for Workaholics, Their Partners and Children and the Clinicians Who Treat Them.* If you or a family member suffers from this disorder, take time to read more about it and get help.

Baby Steps

Now that you have been empowered to make changes in your home and work life, remember that Rome wasn't built in a day. Take baby steps to get things moving in the right direction, but be sure to keep them moving. Taking control of your environment will help you live a happier and healthier life.

The impact that you will have on those around you both at work and at home will be significant. Be careful to stay on track and don't get wrapped up in negativity. Taking charge of your life and becoming more positive at home and at work will make life easier and more enjoyable.

Take a moment to answer the following questions

What is my number one stressor at home?

_____

_____

_____

_____

How can I change my situation or my attitude about this stressor?

_____

_____

_____

_____

How satisfied am I with my job?

_____

_____

_____

_____

If I am not satisfied with my job, what are the reasons?

_____

_____

_____

_____

What do I want to change about my work life?

_____

_____

_____

_____

List the steps that it will take to make these changes:

_____

_____

_____

_____

Overall, how is my work/home life balance? Before you answer this, poll your friends and family.

_____

_____

_____

_____

Step #8

Have Sex Often

The belief that sex is good for the human body is centuries old. Even before we had the medical technology to prove sex was physiologically good for us, the changes in human behavior when a healthy sex life was present are evident. We now know through research that it isn't just about feeling good afterwards, sex has multiple health benefits.

Sex can add to one's ability to stay young and healthy when practiced safely and within the confines of a relationship. On the contrary, promiscuous sex can cause great psychological damage, as well as expose both parties to various sexually transmitted diseases. To maximize the benefits of sex, one must practice it with intimacy, not just as the act itself.

Sex and the Brain

Through the use of positron emission tomography (PET Scan) and fMRI researchers have been able to identify which part of the brain is activated during sexual intercourse. In men the ventral tegmental area (VTA) becomes active; this is the part of the brain that works as a reward center, while the amygdala, the fear center shuts down. This allows a man to get a rush much like that of sky diving.

In women, the VTA is active, but unlike the men, so is the periaqueductal gray matter (PGA). The PGA is part of the fight-or-flight response within the brain. Women basically have a feeling of reward and adrenaline, while men feel rewarded and relaxed.

Rutgers University in New Jersey has proven that romantic love stimulates a different part of the brain system than sex without love. Through the use of the fMRI, we now know that simply viewing a photo of someone that is an intimate relationship can active the VTA portion of the brain and release positive chemicals within the brain. The brains of people in love also tend to show stimulation in the areas of attention and memory recall.

Sex and Immunity

Wilkes University in Pennsylvania found that having intercourse 1-2 times a week raises the level of antibody immunoglobin A (IgA) by as much as a third. The researchers tested saliva from 112 people and divided them into groups of "frequent" and "abstinent", the results were conclusive that those who had sex frequently had much higher antibodies.

IgA is a protein that acts as an antibody by binding to pathogens that enter the body. This process alerts the immune system to attack and destroy the pathogen. Sexual intercourse, when practiced safely, actually helps fight off colds and the flu.

Sex and Cancer

This benefit is geared toward men. Early research showed that frequent ejaculations in men in their 20s meant a significant lower risk for prostate cancer as they got older. A new survey that was released by the National Cancer Institute now shows that middle aged men who average 21 ejaculations in a month have a 33 percent lower risk for prostate cancer, compared to those with only 4-7 ejaculations per month.

Women, on the other hand, increase their risk for cancer if they have multiple partners. Sticking to sex within long term relationships, can actually decrease their risk of contracting the human papilloma virus (HPV) which can change the cells of the cervix and turn cancerous. There is now a vaccine for HPV, but it only protects against 2 types of HPV that cause 70 percent of cervical cancer.

Sex as a Pain Killer

If your spouse complains of a headache, there is good news; sex is actually a good analgesic. During orgasm the brain releases a flood gate of the hormone oxytocin and acts as a natural pain killer. Satisfying sex can decrease arthritis pain, relieve migraine headaches, and reduce overall body aches.

Research also shows that the flow of endorphins can decrease the signs and symptoms of PMS. So, a little love making may actually help keep the peace for a while. Having sex is a great way to relieve pain without the side effects of medicinal painkillers.

Sex for Exercise

Having vigorous sex three times a week for a year is the equivalent calorie burner as walking seventy-five miles. The calories burned are the exact same and total 7,500. If you are into counting calories burned, you can take up to 150 calories for every thirty minutes of intercourse. Not bad for just adding an enjoyable event to your weekly routine.

For women, the benefits of an orgasm can help them later in life. The pelvic muscles get a workout and strengthen during orgasm. Having sex regularly, with an orgasm, may keep them from having urinary incontinence in later years.

Sex Will Make You Happier

The caveat here is that sex makes you happy given that it is taken place in a loving relationship, especially for women. The release of Dehydroepiandrosterone (DHEA) during sex acts as a mood enhancer or natural anti-depressant. Studies show that not only does regular sex reduce anxiety, but good sex has been found to be 10 times more effective than Valium and other medicinal sedatives.

Since sexual intercourse has also been shown to improve sleep, moods are elevated from proper rest. More and more research is showing the link between sex and mood; however, we have known intuitively for years that the lack of sex makes people cranky and less likely to get along with others.

Sex and Longevity

New research proves that the fountain of youth has been right here among us all along. A British study of 1,000 men showed that frequent sex increased lifespan. Of those studied, men who had two or more orgasms a week had half the death rate of those who partook in sex less than once a month.

There are multiple reasons that researchers have been seeing a link between sex and longevity, but most of it goes back to basic science. The chemicals released into the body during sex, especially DHEA, help to repair and heal the tissues of the body. The brain also releases Human Growth Hormone (HGH) during intercourse, helping the body maintain youth. Having quality sex is an important step to living longer and healthier.

Sex for the Heart

In a study that was aimed at identifying sex as a risk factor for stroke in older patients, just the opposite was found. An English study followed 914 men for 20 years and found that not only was there no increased risk for strokes in elderly that have sex, having sex twice a week cut the risk of having a fatal heart attack in half.

Other research studies show that sex increases circulation, reduces blood pressure, and has overwhelming benefits to the heart. Next time you want to do something good for your heart, jump into bed with your partner.

Sex for Hormonal Benefits

Besides the hormones listed above, sexual intercourse is important to the balance of sex hormones testosterone and estrogen. Both are important to men and women, not only for sex drive but for overall health. Having regular sex can help keep these hormones in production and in balance.

Testosterone in men plays a vital role in cardiac health, strong bones, and overall strength. Estrogen in women protects against heart disease, keep her looking young, and enhance mood. New research shows that continuous sexual intercourse helps keep these hormones in balance and increase the benefits they have.

Sex Drive Killers

In an effort to promote healthy sex, it is important to explain some of the things that can kill sex drive. While some problems with libido can be blamed on less than satisfactory relationships, there are many outside factors too. For example, high blood pressure medicine, antidepressants, and other drugs may reduce the drive for sex or render the participant unable to reach orgasm. Anytime you are having sexual dysfunction don't assume that it is your partner, instead talk it over with your doctor to determine the cause.

The everyday hustle and bustle of our busy lives can reduce time for intimacy. Don't let your schedule become so overrun that there is not time for sex. It is easy to let the world get the best of you and your partner get the rest of you, but schedule time to have sex when you are not exhausted. Make time for intimacy and consider it a health requirement.

Foods to Avoid

Some foods can also decrease sex drive. For example, tomatoes contain lycopene and phytofluence which are good for you overall, but decrease testosterone levels. Coconuts are another tricky food, because they increase testosterone, but have an effect on blood vessels that may make arousal difficult.

Food for Better Sex

There are a number of foods that can increase libido and enhance the quality of sex. It seems almost natural that most of these foods are good for you anyway, and you will never find high fat foods on the list.

Watermelon: Contains citrulline which increases blood flow to the genitals. It works like a natural form of Viagra®.

Dark Chocolate: contains serotonin which boosts mood and phenylethylamine, releasing the same chemicals that women get when they are in love. (Little wonder why a box of chocolates is the gift of love)

Asparagus: Rich in folate, increasing histamine. Histamine increases sex drive.

Oysters: If you can stomach them they are a great aphrodisiac for both men and women. They are full of zinc, a vital player in the production of testosterone. They also contain dopamine, a sex drive enhancer.

Pumpkin Seeds: High in zinc, they increase testosterone. Zinc is important to both men and women and is essential for a sex drive. The Omega 3 fatty acids also increase sexual health.

Garlic: The allicin found in garlic helps increase blood flow to sex organs.

Sauerkraut: Packed with healthy compounds, it is no surprise that a 2002 study found that 90 percent of men eating sauerkraut had a significant increase in Libido. The study was published in the Journal of Agricultural and Food Chemistry.

Avocados: Both men and women should eat these regularly because they increase sex drive and stamina.

Bananas: Rich in an enzyme called bromelain, these tasty treats have been proven to increase sex drive in men. The B vitamins are good for both men and women because they boost energy levels during sex.

Beans: The highest on the list of sexual enhancers due to their exceptionally high levels of zinc.

Broccoli: This is a tricky one because it is great for sex drive in men, but has the opposite effect in women.

Celery: Eating celery raw increases the pheromones released by men. Women will actually be aroused by the perspiration of men who consume celery.

Chilies: Have a chemical called capsaicin which increases blood flow and enhances mood by releasing endorphins.

Eggs: Help regulate testosterone and estrogen

Fish: Enhance the nervous system and boost circulation, increasing the quality of sex.

Nuts: Full of fatty acids that are essential to the production of hormones, they also contain L-Arginine which enhances erections. Even the smell of almonds, can help arouse a women, while pine nuts are good for sperm quality. Overall, nuts have multiple sex benefits.

Nutmeg: This is a long time libido booster used in Indian medicine. Studies show that very small doses of nutmeg can have the same effects as Viagra®.

Soy: In women this acts as a natural hormone booster. However, women with a history of breast cancer should avoid it.

Steak: Boosts testosterone and increases the urge to have sex.

Sex is a Need

Many people view sexual intercourse as a want, when in fact it is a need. The human body was designed to partake in sex and do so frequently. The research is conclusive that having sex has many benefits and can help you live longer. Increase your mood, your health, and your relationships through regular intercourse.

The following charts will help you identify if you are having good quality sex often. Life can be so busy that we may think we are having sex more often than we actually are. Track your sexual patterns for one month to see if you are getting enough to reap the health benefits.

Orgasm Chart – Week One

	YES	NO	LENGTH OF TIME
MONDAY			
TUESDAY			
WEDNESDAY			
THURSDAY			
FRIDAY			
Saturday			
Sunday			

Orgasm Chart – Week Two

	YES	NO	LENGTH OF TIME
MONDAY			
TUESDAY			
WEDNESDAY			
THURSDAY			
FRIDAY			
Saturday			
Sunday			

Orgasm Chart – Week Three

	YES	NO	LENGTH OF TIME
MONDAY			
TUESDAY			
WEDNESDAY			
THURSDAY			
FRIDAY			
Saturday			
Sunday			

Orgasm Chart – Week Four

	YES	NO	LENGTH OF TIME
MONDAY			
TUESDAY			
WEDNESDAY			
THURSDAY			
FRIDAY			
Saturday			
Sunday			

Step #9

Sleep Your Way to a Younger You

You may be asking how we can devote and entire chapter to the importance of sleep. It seems like a common sense topic, but the impact of not getting enough sleep and the right kind of sleep can have devastating consequences on the human body. Sleep is a necessity for normal bodily function and is a necessary function for both psychological and physiological health.

Missing a little sleep here and there is not nearly as damaging as long term sleep deprivation, but it should still be avoided if at all possible. Sleep should be viewed as a necessity and not a luxury. Society has embraced the technology boom, but the human body is taking a beating for it. The 24/7 work day doesn't allow the brain a chance to recharge, leaving millions of people at risk for health problems, both physically and emotionally.

The number of hours a person needs for sleep is dependent on many factors, one of which is age. An infant requires as much as 16 hours of sleep in order to grow and develop normally. Teenagers should get about 9, while adults need between 7-8 hours to function at full capacity. Over the past 40 years, there has been a significant change in the amount of sleep that Americans have been getting. While adults averaged 8.5 hours per night in 1960, recent research shows that they now average only about 7, which means an 18% reduction. Over time, this adds up to thousands of missed hours of sleep.

The Lack of Sleep

Maybe the most recognized side effect of sleep deprivation is a decrease in mental functions. Learning and memory are greatly reduced when people do not get a good night of sleep. The brain needs to rest in order for it to absorb new information. While the body is resting, memories are consolidated, thus making room for new information. In one study, participants were given information to remember. Half of the study group was deprived of REM sleep, while the other half was allowed to follow normal sleep patterns. The group that was not allowed REM sleep could not remember the information, whereas the control group had no trouble remembering.

As more of society is lacking sleep, they are also increasing their waist size. Sleeping is a vital part of maintaining a proper weight because it allows the body to process carbohydrates and also helps maintain proper levels of hormones that are responsible for appetite control. The University of Chicago conducted a study on sleep and obesity. They found that subjects that slept for 4 hours a night for two nights in a row had a change in hormone levels. Leptin, a hormone that tells the brain that it is full, was decreased by 18%. Ghrelin, a hormone that triggers hunger was increased 28%. These hormones were only discovered in the last ten years, but researchers have found that their balance is necessary for proper weight maintenance.

Much of our focus has been about internal dangers of sleep deprivation, but external dangers can be deadly. A lack of sleep causes a decrease of safety and inability to perform tasks properly. Some of the more horrific accidents in history have been linked to sleep deprivation in employees. Two nuclear disasters: Chernobyl and Three Mile Island, as well as the Exxon Val Dez oil tanker and the explosion of the Challenger were all linked to errors made from sleep deprived employees. These may be extreme examples, but new studies show that the simple act of driving without adequate sleep can be even more dangerous than driving while intoxicated.

Less dangerous, but not without consequence, is the effect that the lack of sleep can have on mood. Impatience and irritability can become part of everyday life, therefore driving away the people you love. The American Academy of Sleep Medicine has concluded that there is a direct correlation between sleep quality and relationship quality in both men and women. It would not be too far of a stretch to say longer and higher quality sleep can help interpersonal relationships with your spouse, children, and co-workers.

Even if you chose to remain grumpy and moody, you may want to consider getting more sleep for the sake of your heart. Not getting enough sleep has been proven to lead to high blood pressure, heart disease, and irregular heartbeats. The University of Chicago found that a lack in sleep can increase calcium build-up in the main arteries of the heart, which in turn can cause plaque to break off, leading to heart attack and strokes. The study showed that as little as one hour a night less of sleep can increase coronary calcium by 16%.

If you can find the time to squeeze in a nap during the day, it may save your life. The Harvard School of Public Health studied 23,000 adults and found that those who took a nap during the day had a 37% less chance of dying from a heart attack. Those that had occasional naps lowered their risk by 12%. While the study did not state to do so, we recommend our patients with known heart diseases to make napping part of their regular routine. Along with high cholesterol and other risk factors, sleep deprivation is becoming a recognized red flag for predicting heart disease.

If vanity is your weakness, then maybe the body's need for beauty sleep may convince you. The body repairs cells and tissues while we sleep, helping maintain a youthful outward appearance.   When you skip sleep, your body is unable to properly manage endocrine function, which in turn speeds up the clock and causes premature aging. Not only will the appearance of aging be more noticeable, age related illnesses will be more likely to occur.

In one study, patients were deprived of sleep and then their ability to regulate blood sugar levels was checked. At the height of sleep deprivation, subjects took up to 40% more time to process glucose. Basically, sleep deprivation put them in a state that mimicked Type II diabetes, a condition that is known to affect multiple organ systems. This study along with others, have lead researchers to understand that sleep deprivation has consequences that damage overall health.

Many times when we see patients that have a cold or recurrent sinus infection, they also have been overworked and not getting adequate rest. It has long been recognized by the medical community that sleep affects the immune system. New research shows that missing sleep actually increases the body's trigger for inflammation, thus causing the body to fight off or attack its own tissue. Many diseases, including heart disease, arthritis, and some cancers are a result of an inflammatory process. The American Academy of Sleep Medicine published a study that found each hour of sleep deprivation reported by patients in a study correlated with an 8% increase in CRP (C - reactive protein) and a 7% increase in interleukin-6 (IL-6), both of which are responsible for inflammation within the body.

Sleep is also is necessary for the production and function of the body's T-cells, which are necessary for fighting off cancer. James McClain from The National Cancer Institute studied women over a ten year period and found that getting less than 7 hours of sleep increases the risk of cancer. Other studies have shown that increased exercise without adequate sleep actually cancels out the cancer fighting benefits of exercise.

The bottom line on sleep is that we need it not only for optimal health, but for basic function. It not only controls how we look on the outside, but how we operate on the inside. Without adequate sleep, the body is destined for not only short-term consequences, but long-term health problems. On the contrary, getting a good amount of quality sleep can keep you beautiful and healthy.

How Sleep Works

Our bodies sleep in a cycle that is known as the circadian rhythm, which is made up of important stages. Each stage is important to proper brain function and homeostasis of the entire body. Getting enough sleep and the right kind of sleep is required for good health.

Stage 1, also called light sleep is when the body first drifts off. During this stage the body can be easily awakened by sounds, smells, and temperature changes. The brain may see flashes of images as it begins to power down as eyes move slowly and muscles start to relax. Many people have experienced a falling sensation, twitch, or may be suddenly startled in this stage.

In *Stage 2*, the eye movement stops and brain waves become slower. Occasionally the brain may have bursts of energy, called sleep spindles, which can be seen on an EEG. Heart rate decreases and body temperature drops during this time. About half of our sleep is spent in stage 2 sleep.

By *Stage 3*, Delta waves (very slow waves) begin to appear. This is the stage that transitions the body from light sleep to deep sleep.

As the body falls into a deep sleep, *Stage 4* brings on a constant flow of Delta waves. This is the part of sleep where bed-wetting or sleep walking usually take place.

The last stage of sleep, *Stage 5* is often referred to as REM (Rapid Eye Movement) sleep. The first occurrence of REM usually starts after 90 minutes and lasts only a short time. As the body continues to cycle through the circadian rhythm, each REM sleep section becomes longer until it lasts about an hour. During REM, the muscles are temporarily paralyzed so that the body is prevented from acting out dreams. While the brain increases activity, the muscles are in a completely relaxed state. REM sleep stimulates the part of the brain that is used for learning and REM plays a significant role in memory and cognitive functions, as well as other physiological functions of the body.

During REM sleep the body is unable to regulate temperature, so sleeping in a room that is not too hot or too cold will keep the body from disrupting deep sleep in order to get comfortable. If you remember waking from a deep sleep feeling cold or sweating, you were probably in REM sleep. Waking up from that sleep disrupts much needed brain activity.

Falling and Staying Asleep

The days seem to be filled with constant chaos. Moving from one meeting to another, interruptions, stress, and high energy all make it harder to wind down at night. Getting to sleep and staying asleep is a problem for some of our patients, but some simple tips listed below may help.

- Take time to decompress. Watch television or read a book while to take your mind off of the events of the day.

- Limit your caffeine intake. Depending on your sensitivity, you may want to stop all caffeine as early as noon, but no later than 5pm.

- Keep your room at a comfortable temperature. Cool, but not cold, is best for optimal sleep.

- Covers should keep you warm, but make sure they are not too heavy or cause you to get tangled, both of which will wake you up at night.

- A hot cup of herbal tea or warm milk will help put your body in sleep mode.

- Never go to bed angry. This will disrupt your circadian rhythm. Ladies – this will also cause wrinkles!

- Sleep in total darkness. New research shows a link between sleeping with a light on at night and a decrease in melatonin levels, thus causing an increase in the risk for cancer.

- Make a conscious effort to relax your jaw before falling asleep. This will help prevent jaw pain and teeth grinding.

- Be sure that your mattress is comfortable, yet firm. Doing so will prevent back pain.

- Aroma therapy can be helpful. Lavender is a good scent that promotes a good night sleep.

- Sleep in silence.

A Word on Snoring

Snoring is not just a noisy and annoying problem; it can have real health consequences. It is caused by the tissue in the back of your throat vibrating when air is moving from the mouth and nose to the lungs. Snoring can disrupt sleep patterns because a person may wake themselves up. In some cases, snoring is a sign of obstructive sleep apnea, a serious problem where the patient stops breathing during sleep. The lack of oxygen to the brain can greatly increase the risk for heart attack and stroke.

Patients who snore should have a sleep study to determine the seriousness of their snoring. There are many ways to treat snoring which include C-PAP machines which force continuous air in through a face mask, pillar procedures which keep the tissue from obstructing the airway through the insertion of small posts in the back of the throat, or by using an oral appliance that will reposition the jaw. Not all solutions are right for everyone, but after a sleep study your doctor can help you decide which is best for you.

Overall, the importance of good sleep can't be stressed enough. The right amount of sleep, in the right environment, with the highest quality of deep sleep will help prevent disease and lead to a healthier body, mind, and spirit.

In an effort to track your own sleep habits and heighten awareness of ways to improve it, take a moment to look at your sleep patterns.

	SNORE?	HOURS SLEPT	QUALITY OF SLEEP
MONDAY			
TUESDAY			
WEDNESDAY			
THURSDAY			
FRIDAY			
Saturday			
Sunday			

You may need to ask your spouse, but document whether you experienced any snoring during sleep. If the answer is yes, discuss with your physician the possibility of getting a sleep study.

Step #10

Have Fun and Enjoy Life

F un is defined by anything that takes you away from the pressures and responsibilities of life. It is a mini vacation from reality. Fun is not only desirable, it is a necessity to good health. Our bodies were made to laugh and enjoy life, not to be serious all the time. Serious people die young (and miserable). The old saying that miserable people live forever, simply isn't true. It may feel like they never die, but if you look at those that have lived to be 100 years of age, they are generally the people who kept a good sense of humor and a realistic perspective on the trials and tribulations of life.

Years ago, Norman Cousins wrote a book, which later became a movie, about how he survived a devastating diagnosis through the use of laughter. In his book *The Anatomy of an Illness*, he describes how watching old Charlie Chaplin movies spurred him to better health. Prior to him coming forward and sharing his story, few people realized the importance of laughter in the body's ability to heal. However, the past 30 years have been filled with new research and scientific evidence that laughter, fun, and leisure activities are not only important to healing, they are essential to disease prevention.

The Research on Fun

Drs. Lee Berk and Stanley Tan of Loma Linda University Medical Center of California studied the effects of humor on the body. Their research now proves that laughing has physiological benefits to the body. Patients who laugh have the benefits of lower blood pressure, reduced stress, and increased immune systems.

At the University of Maryland School of Medicine, Dr. Michael Miller studied the effects of humor on heart health. Through a research study at the University, they subjected 20 healthy patients to two movies, *Saving Private Ryan* (a serious war movie) and *Kingpin* (a comedy). Those that watched the war movie showed a decreased blood flow of 35 percent while those that watched the comedy showed an increase in blood flow by 22 percent. The results solidified that laughter is good medicine for the heart!

In line with the studies in Maryland, Duke University published a study on the effects of depression on heart patients. Dr. Wei Jiang studied 1,000 patients with heart failure. Those that suffered mild depression were 44 percent more likely to die. Both of these studies were presented at the American College of Cardiology meeting and were shown to be significant to the health and wellness of heart patients.

Patients who suffer chronic pain are more likely to have a higher quality of life if they are subjected to humor. Laughing produces endorphins that act like natural pain killers within the body. Humor has been used for years in children's hospitals and is now making its way into mainstream adult medicine. Many hospitals are recognizing the benefits of humor and offering more comedy channels on the in-room televisions. Doctors are also encouraging more "fun" in the lives of their patients.

Having a good old time is good for the body, as well as the mind, and is essential to healthy relationships. Laughing with your family and friends creates bonds in a physiological way. When you make memories and develop feelings about those you are with, the brain keeps a file on the event. If you have files that are "happy", you will want to spend more time with that person. This is a subconscious process. The body recognizes the person, identifies with the previous memories, and then responds. This is why we get butterflies or the opposite sick feeling in our stomach when we are in the company of others.

Because laughter and relaxation are so important, family vacations are at the heart of bonding and building relationships, while preserving one's own sanity. A heart disease prevention trial completed at the State University of New York at Oswego looked at the vacation habits of 12,000 men ages 35-57. The results were astounding and showed a major link between heart disease and work habits. Men who took the time to vacation once a year reduced their overall death rate by 20 percent and risk of heart disease by as much as 30 percent. The relationship between workaholism and heart disease was clear and showed that those men who did not vacation for the past 5 years had the highest risk of heart disease.

A Framingham Heart Study also showed a link between coronary heart disease and women who do not take vacation. In that study, women who took a vacation every 6 years or less were 8 times more likely to develop coronary artery disease or have a heart attack.

Vacations and relaxation are also linked to prevention of cancer, diabetes, and a number of other diseases. The lack of laughter has a domino effect: stress leads to physiological effects like increased waist size and belly fat, which is associated with diabetes and heart disease, which in turn lead to failing health and ultimately death. The opposite is also true: increasing the fun in your life leads to reduced stress, which leads to better circulation, which leads to healthy muscles and brain function, etc.

Fun Blockers

Over the last several decades, people have become very serious and seem to have forgotten how to laugh. They not only forgot how to laugh with friends about external humorous events, they seem to have forgotten how to laugh at themselves. This change in our culture has sent many people into a downward spiral of depression.

In an effort to learn how to laugh, we should explore, and debunk, the barriers that keep us from having fun. Many of these excuses have also been listed in Lance Armstrong's Live Strong workbook.

- Lack of time – this is simply the most ridiculous of all the excuses and reasons that we have ever hear. You can do the same amount of work in the same amount of time and incorporate humor and a good spirit.

- I take my job seriously – Good for you! We are glad you do, but you don't have to work 24/7. Taking yourself too seriously can be detrimental to your health and your mental wellbeing. You really are not as important as you think you are and you don't control the universe. Relax, as soon as you understand that concept, your life will improve.

- I don't know how – Really? We are born to be inquisitive and to explore our world. Everyone has a different definition of fun. If you don't know your definition, spend some time finding out who you are and what you like. Take up a few hobbies until one sticks.

- Lack of Money – This may come as a surprise, but fun can be as cheap or as expensive as you make it. The more creative you are, the cheaper it is. In many cases – it's free!

Fun Ideas

As stated earlier, fun is not defined the same for everyone. Finding what you enjoy in life can be a bit of a challenge for some and very simple for others. In an effort to boost your creative juices, below is a list of ideas help incorporate fun back into your life.

- Have family game night. This may sound corny, but break out the old board games once a month and gather around the table after dinner. If the kids are older, try poker or other strategy games.

- Go for a walk in the dark. Take a flashlight and go for a long walk. The brisk night air will make for a good night sleep, but even better could be the conversations that spontaneously erupt between you and your walking partner.

- Camp out in the back yard. If you are not up for an all-nighter, try just having a picnic or roasting marshmallows in an outdoor fire pit.

- Have a family talent show. Believe it or not, this can be so much fun, and a bundle of laughs.

- Take a spontaneous trip with a friend. Decide on Thursday where to go for the weekend. You can find great last minute deals and the adventurous spirit will make you feel young again.

- Take an art class. Even if you only draw stick figures. Allowing the other side of your brain to take over for a while will aid in the reduction of stress.

- Rent some classic funny movies. Sometimes half the fun is just looking back at the old styles and hairdos of the past.

- Have a girl or guys night out. Stay out of trouble, but share a few laughs and reminisce over the good old days.

- Do something out of the ordinary. Vacationing on the coast? Take a shrimp boat out and see what they catch. You have to pay a fee to "ride along" but it is a unique adventure.

- Ask the family to all write poems about the family. Be careful – you may have to learn to laugh at yourself on this one.

- Make a treasure chest and fill it with items that your pirate will love. Then make a map and let them use your clues to find it. You will have fun doing it and they will have fun finding it.

- Take ballroom dancing lessons. This is a great way to get into shape while having fun.

- Have a dinner party with a theme. Regardless of your theme, conversation among guests should bring a few good laughs.

- Join a progressive dinner for eight (or ten). This is where everyone travels from house to house trying each other's food.

- Go to a sporting event. It is hard to be miserable with thousand of happy people around you.

Whatever you come up with, remember that the key is to take a mini vacation from the realities of life. Finding your joy of life once again will keep you healthy and make for a much happier journey through this thing we call life.

Take a moment to list the things that you have enjoyed doing in the past. These may be things like: golf, dancing, chess, playing an instrument, etc.

_____

_____

_____

_____

_____

Look at the list above and see which of these you would like to do again. List them below:

_____

_____

_____

_____

_____

Make a list of the 10 things you would like to do before you die. This "bucket list" (things you must do before you kick the bucket) will help keep you involved in things that you find interesting. Find a way to start accomplishing the things listed below. If you finish before you die, make another list!

1 _____

2 _____

3 _____

4 _____

5 _____

6 _____

7 _____

8 _____

9 _____

10 _____

Conclusion

Now is your chance to put this 10 step program into place. You can add years to your life while improving your quality of life very quickly and easily. For the most part, there isn't anything magical about this program; it is simply about bringing us back to the basics of life and living. Happiness and wellness are often found in the simplicities of life and in our natural resources.

With a combination of almost 80 years as health professionals, we have seen people make choices that will either add to their life or take away from it. We are glad to see that you are being proactive and are ready to make changes that will help you live a longer life, with many "younger" years. Your decision will affect not only you, but those around you.

Your choice to live a healthier lifestyle will greatly impact those that you love. Congratulations on being a positive influence and good luck!

Six Month Follow-Up

It has been six months since you decided to take the steps to becoming a younger you. In an effort to make this program successful, there has to be accountability. What changes have you made in your life? Of those, which ones had the most positive impact? Go through the steps below and make comments. This process will help you focus on what you have accomplished and what areas you still need to work on.

Step #1 Know Your Family History

Did you record accurate information within this section of the book? ___Yes ___No

Has anything significant happened since you first made the recordings? ___Yes ___No If so, go back and add them now.

Did you give a copy of your family history to your siblings and children? ___Yes ___No If not, do so within the next week.

Step #2 Know Your Health Status

Did you have a physical exam with your doctor? ___Yes ___No

Did you record the findings? ___Yes ___No

What is your current weight? _____

How has your Body Mass (BMI) Index changed? ___Yes ___No

Are you at a healthy weight? ___Yes ___No

What is your Body Mass Index? _____

Weight in Pounds

		120	130	140	150	160	170	180	190	200	210	220	230	240	250
	4'6	29	31	34	36	39	41	43	46	48	51	53	56	58	60
	4'8	27	29	31	34	36	38	40	43	45	47	49	52	54	56
	4'10	25	27	29	31	34	36	38	40	42	44	46	48	50	52
	5'0	23	25	27	29	31	33	35	37	39	41	43	45	47	49
	5'2	22	24	26	27	29	31	33	35	37	38	40	42	44	46
	5'4	21	22	24	26	28	29	31	33	34	36	38	40	41	43
	5'6	19	21	23	24	26	27	29	31	32	34	36	37	39	40
	5'8	18	20	21	23	24	26	27	29	30	32	34	35	37	38
	5'10	17	19	20	22	23	24	26	27	29	30	32	33	35	36
	6'0	16	18	19	20	22	23	24	26	27	28	30	31	33	34
	6'2	15	17	18	19	21	22	23	24	26	27	28	30	31	32
	6'4	15	16	17	18	20	21	22	23	24	26	27	28	29	30
	6'6	14	15	16	17	19	20	21	22	23	24	25	27	28	29
	6'8	13	14	15	17	18	19	20	21	22	23	24	25	26	28

Height in Feet and Inches

■ Healthy Weight   ■ Overweight   ■ Obese

Note: This chart is for adults aged 20 years and older. Source: U.S. Surgeon General

If you had any abnormal findings, did you follow-up on them?

_____Yes _____No

What tests have you not completed that you need to still complete?

_____

_____

_____

Step #3: Modify Your Eating Habits

What changes have you made to your diet?_____

What changes do you still want to make to your diet plan? _____

_____

List below the steps you are going to take to put these changes into action:

_____

_____

_____

_____

Step#4: Go to the Spa

Have you taken time to go to the spa? ___Yes ___No

Make a list of how you feel after a spa treatment:

_____

_____

_____

_____

Step #5: Adopt an Exercise Program

List the simple changes you have made over the last 6 months that have increased your activity level:

_____

_____

_____

_____

Have you adopted an exercise program? ___Yes ___No

Does your program have cardio components? ___Yes ___No

Does your program have strengthening components?

___Yes ___No

Does your program have components that increase flexibility?
___Yes ___No

Step #6: Get Spiritually Centered

Have you adopted a daily routine of prayer or meditation?
___Yes ___No

Have you increased your activity within your social or spiritual circles? ___Yes ___No

Make a list of other ways you have been able to increase your spirituality:

_____

_____

_____

_____

_____

Make a list of things that you still want to accomplish:

_____

_____

_____

_____

_____

Step #7: Take Control of Your Work and Home Life

Look back at your number one stressor at home. Has it improved in the last 6 months? ___Yes ___No

How has your attitude changed in the last 6 months and what things could you still do to change? _____

Are you in your same job as 6 months ago? ___Yes ___No

Are you happier? ___Yes ___No

List the ways that you have found balance in home and work life:

_____

_____

_____

_____

Step#8: Have Sex Often

Take a moment to record your sexual activity again. When you are done, see if you have improved since 6 months ago.

Orgasm Chart – Sixth Month Comparison

	YES	NO	LENGTH OF TIME
MONDAY			
TUESDAY			
WEDNESDAY			
THURSDAY			
FRIDAY			
Saturday			
Sunday			

Step #9: Sleep Your Way to a Younger You

What steps have you taken to better your sleep patterns?

_____

_____

_____

_____

Record your sleep again below. Has it improved?

	SNORE?	HOURS SLEPT	QUALITY OF SLEEP
MONDAY			
TUESDAY			
WEDNESDAY			
THURSDAY			
FRIDAY			
Saturday			
Sunday			

Step #10: Have Fun and Enjoy Life

Look at your Bucket List. Have you checked any of these items off?

_____

What hobbies have you taken up over the last 6 months?

_____

Do you have any new interests? _____ If so, list how you are going to incorporate those interests into your schedule.

_____

_____

_____

_____

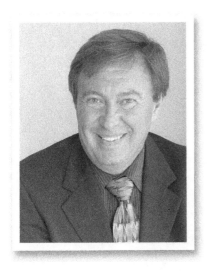

Walter Gaman, MD

Dr. Gaman is Board Certified in Family Practice in both the United States and Canada. He received his medical degree from the University of Manitoba and is a member of the Texas Medical Association, Texas Academy of Family Physicians, The American Academy of Family Physicians, the American Medical Association, and the Canadian College of Family Physicians (President, Manitoba Chapter, 1981).

Dr. Gaman was named one of America's Top Family Doctors for 2002-2003 by the Consumers Research Council of America. The Fort Worth Business Press has named him one of their Healthcare Heroes of 2005 and later he was also voted one of the "Best Doctors in Dallas" by D Magazine.

Dr. Gaman has helped many people reach ultimate health and continues to focus on preventative and proactive medicine. When not seeing patients, he can be seen and heard as an expert in the media. He is often consulted on corporate wellness and has been known to help top executives and high profile individuals from all over the world reach optimum health and performance.

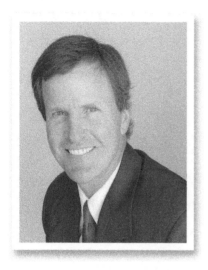

J. Mark Anderson, MD

A Dallas native, Dr. Anderson did his undergraduate work at Texas A&M University and received his medical degree from the University of Texas Medical Branch-Galveston. He completed residency training in Family Medicine at Southwestern Medical School and St. Paul Medical Center in Dallas, Texas. He is currently Board Certified in Family Medicine. He is a member of the Texas Medical Association, Texas Academy of Family Physicians, and The American Academy of Family Physicians.

Dr. Anderson often speaks to large groups on a number of topics. He appears within the media as an expert on proactive health and wellness and has become a household name to many.

Dr. Anderson has helped thousands, including professional athletes and high profile individuals, reach ultimate health. Through his medical practice he continues his passion to help others stay young and active. This is why he was voted one of the "Best Doctors in Dallas" by D Magazine.

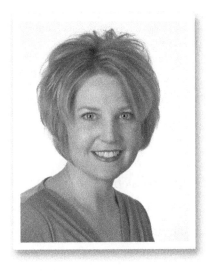

Judy Gaman

As a published author and public speaker, Judy has been entertaining and educating audiences for years. She received her degree in health sciences, with a concentration in clinical research administration from the prestigious George Washington University School of Medicine and Health Sciences. She has over 20 years of experience within the medical field.

As an award winning author, she has found that writing is another way to impact people and be a positive force in their lives. Her writing has also lead to multiple opportunities to speak to groups both large and small, and her presentations have empowered a menagerie of people from CEOs to stay at home moms.

References

Preamble

Harvard University (2002) Harvard Health Newsletter. February 2002

Robinson, B. (2007) Chained to the Desk: A Guide for Workaholics, Their Partners and children and the Clinicians Who Treat Them (2nd ed.) NYU Press

Anderson, J.(2005) Report Highlights Gap Between European and Us Vacation Time. Ergoweb. May 2005

Crandon, B. Health Matters: Computer Work Can Strain Eyes: Follow Some Simple Suggestions To Reduce Computer Induced Eye Strain. Retrieved October 20, 2009 from http://oldkcsmall.biz

Step #1

National Cancer Inst 2009 July 15; 101(14): 984-92

National Cancer Institute. US National Institute on Health. www.cancer.gov

Centers for Disease Control and Prevention (CDC) www.cdc.gov

Stanford School of Medicine. Understanding Genetics When Genetics Go Bad: Mutations and Disease. Retrieved on October 15, 2009 from http://www.thetech.org/genetics/art04_bad.php

Rowland, B., Frey, R. (2005) "Ulcers, Digestive" Gale Encyclopedia of Alternative Medicine. The Gale Group, Inc. 2005

BBC News (2007) Heart Disease Genetic Link Found. http://new.bbc.co.uk

Adams, J. (2008) Pharmacogenomics and Personalized Medicine.

Nature Education 1(1)

Alzheimer's Research Trust (2009) Largest Ever Alzheimer's Gene Study Unveils Dementia Mysteries. Nature Genetics, Vol. 41, No 10. October 06, 2009. Pp1088-1093

Burger, J (2006) Biochips Tools of the 21st Century Medicine. PMID: 16553220

http://familyhistory.hhs.gov

Step #2

Http://www.nlm.nih.gov/medlineplus/laboratorytests.html

http://www.fda.gov

http://labtestsonline.org (Developed by the American Association of Clinical Chemistry)

Step #3

WebMD. Health & Cooking. How to Read a Nutritional Label. Retrieved on November 1, 2009 from http://www.webmd.com/food-recipes/features/how-read-nutritional-label.com

Wallinga, D., Sorensen, J., (et al) (2009) Not so Sweet: Missing Mercury and High Fructose Corn Syrup. Institute for Agriculture and Trade Policy (IATP) January 26, 2009

SixWise.com (2006) 12 Dangerous Food Additives. The Dirty Dozen Foods Additives You Really Need to be Aware of. Six Wise Newsletter April 5, 2006

Fujioka, K, Greenway, F., Sheard, J., Ying, Y. (2006) The Effects of Grapefruit on Weight and Insulin Resistance: Relationship to the Metabolic Syndrome. Journal of Medicinal Food 9 Spring 2006: 49-54

FEBS Lett., August 1998 433 (1-2): 44-46

Mattes, Rd, (et al.) (2008) Impact of Peanuts and Tree Nuts on Body

Weight and healthy Weight Loss in Audults. Journal of Nutrition. 138 (17415-17455)

De Olivera, M., Sichieri, R., Sanchez Moura, A., (2003) Nutrition. 19: 253-256

Hlebowicz, J., (2009) Blood Glucose Response in Relation to Gastric Emptying and Satiety in Healthy Subjects. Appetite, Vol. 53, Issue 2, October 2009 p 249-252

Biochemical and Biophysical Research Communications

Volume 374, Issue 3, 26 September 2008, Pages 431-436

Tubelius, P., Stan, V., Zachrisson, A., (2005) Increasing Work-place Healthiness with the Probiotic Lactobacillus Reuteri: a Randomized, Double Blind, Placebo Controlled Study. Enviro Health 2005 Nov 7; 4:25

Step #4

http://www.therapeuticpresence.com/history.html

Archives of Internal Medicine, Vol. 166, No. 22, December 11, 2006

Complementary Therapies in Clinical Practice. Vol. 15, Issue 2, May 2009, p 119

Publix Greenwise Market Magazine. All You Need is Love. February 2008

Step #5

Lee, I. M. (2003) Physical Activity and Cancer Prevention – Data from Epidemiologic Studies. Medicine & Science in Sports and Exercise, 35 (11), 1823-1827

Centers for Disease Control and Prevention. (2007) Overweight and obesity: Health Consequences. Retrieved on October 15, 2009 from www.cdc.gov/nccdphp/dnpa/pbesity/index.htm

Cancer Epidemiol Biomarkers. Prevention, 2008 July: 17(7); 1714-

http://www.hhs.gov

Journal of Lipid Research August 2009

http://www.americanheart.org

Jacobs, D, Pereira, M (2004) Physical Activity Relative Body Weight and Risk of Death among Women. New England Journal of Medicine. Volume 351:2753-2755. December 23, 2004

Panning, J. (2000) Mental Health Benefits of Exercise. Mental Health Journal. Retrieved on October 30, 2009 from http://www.findcounseling.com/journal/health-fitness/

Merritt, R. (2006) Exercise Fights Depression. Retrieved on November 1, 2009 from http://hdlighthouse.org/see/diet/triad/exercise/duke.htm

Neuromolecular Medicine. Vol. 10 No. 2 June 2008. P47-58

Internal Journal of Clinical Practice. Vol. 63 Issue 2, p303-320

http://www.surgeongeneral.gov

Arthritis and Rheumatism (2007) 57(3), p 407-414

Wiley-Blackwell (2008) Exercise Program Improves Symptoms of Arthritis Patients. Science Daily. January 9, 2009

Brown University News Release (2001) Diet and Exercise Cut Type 2 Diabetes Risk Drastically, Study Finds. August 8, 2001

British Journal of Sports Medicine (2007) 41:649-655

Fred Hutchison Research Center Press Release. Moderate Physical Activity is Critical for Reducing the Risk of Chronic Disease in Men and Women. Released June 11, 2007

Nieman, D. (1995) Can Exercise Each Day Keep Cancer at Bay? The Free Library. Retrieved on November 28, 2009 from http://www.thefreelibrary.com/canexerciseeachdaykeepcanceratbay?-a016728278

Penedo, F. Dahn, J. (2005) Exercise and Well-Being Associated with

Physical Activity: Physical Health and Benefits of Physical Activity. Current Opinion Psychiatry. 2005; 18(2): 189-193

Step #6

www.who.int

Religious People Live Longer Than Non-believers. Retrieved on November 15, 2009 from http://webmd.com/news/20000809/religious-people-live-longer-than-nonbelievers

Newburg, A., Walderman, M. (2009) How God Changes Your Brain. Ballantine Books

Davidson, RJ, Kabat-Zinn, J., et al (2003)Alterations in Brain and Immune Function Produced by Mindful Meditation. Psychosomatic Medicine. Vol. 65 p 564-570

Step #7

Studies Show a Sunny Ooutlook for Health, Longer Life (2009) www.Mayoclinic.org/news July 22, 2009

Beck, M (2009) Health Matters: Starting to Feel Older? New Study Show Attitude Can be Critical. Wall Street Journal. October 17, 2009. Retrieved on November 1, 2009 from

http://online.wsj.com/article/SB10001424052748704471504574445263666118226.html

Goetzel, RZ., Anderson, Dr., et al (1998) The Relationship Between Modifiable Health Risks and Health Expenditure: An Analysis of the Multi-power HERO health Risks and Cost Database. Journal of Occupational Environmental Medicine. Vol. 40: 843-854

Working Hard of Harly Working? Research Studies Effects on Job Simplification on Employee Productivity. September 17, 2007. Retrieved on November 1, 2009 from http://www.physorg.com/news109260517.html

Robinson, B. (2001) Chained to the Desk: A Guidebook for Worka-holics, Their Partners and the children and the Clinicians Who Treat Them. (1st Ed.) NYU Press

Step #8

Fisher H, A Aron and LL Brown(2005) Romantic Love: An fMRI study of a neural mechanism for mate choice. Journal of Comparative Neurology, 493:58-62. 2005

A Aron, HE Fisher, DJ Mashek, G Strong, HF Li, and LL Brown (2005) Reward, Motivation and Emotion Systems Associated with Early-Stage Intense Romantic Love: an fMRI study. Journal of Neurophysiology 94:327-337

Doheny, K. (2008) "10 Surprising Health Benefits of Sex," WebMD (reviewed by Chang, L., M.D.)

Ebrahim, S., May, M., et al (2002) Sexual Intercourse and Risk of Ischemic Stroke and Coronary Heart Disease: The Caerphilly Study. Epidemiol Community Health 2002; 56:99-102

Charnetski CJ, Brennan FX. Sexual frequency and salivary immu-noglobulin A (IgA). Psychological Reports 2004 Jun;94(3 Pt 1):839-44. Data on length of relationship and sexual satisfaction were not related to the group differences.

Giles, GG et al. Sexual factors and prostate cancer. British Journal of Urology International. August 2003. 92(3): 211-216.

"Sauerkraut is Newest Celebrity Superfood; Fremont Finds Recent Nutritionist Studies Fuel Adoption". Business Wire. FindArticles.com. 1 Dec, 2009. http://findarticles.com/p/articles/mi_m0EIN/is_2005_June_15/ai_n13815284/

Step #9

National Sleep Foundation. 2001 "Sleep in America" Poll. Washington, DC: National Sleep Foundation; 2001.

Spiegel, K., Tasali, E., Penev, P., Van Cauter, E. (2004) Brief communication: sleep curtailment in healthy young men is associated with decreased leptin levels, elevated ghrelin levels, and increased hunger and appetite. Ann Intern Med. 141: 846–850.

Park, A. (2008) Lack of Sleep Linked to Heart Problems. Time.com December 23, 2008

The Science of Sleep. Retrieved on November 2, 2009 from http://www.bbc.co.uk/science/humanbody/sleep/articles/whatissleep.shtml

Shmidt, H. (2002) Deadly Combination. Psychiatric News September 20, 2002

Volume 37 Number 18 Page 28

Siesta in Healthy Adults and Coronary Mortality in the General Population

Arch Intern Med, Feb 2007; 167: 296 - 301.

Patel SR; Zhu X; Storfer-Isser A; Mehra R; Jenny NS; Tracy R; Redline S. Sleep duration and biomarkers of inflammation. SLEEP 2009;32(2):200-204.

McClain J, et al, "Association between physical activity, sleep duration, and cancer risk among women in Washington County, MD: a prospective cohort study" AACR 2008 Abstract B145.

Step#10

Cousins, N (2005) Anatomy of an Illness as Perceived by the Patient. WW Norton & Co.

American Physiological Society (2009, April 17). Laughter Remains Good Medicine. Science Daily. Retrieved December 12, 2009

University of Maryland Medical Center (2005) University of Maryland School of Medicine Study shows Laughter Helps Blood Vessels Function Better. Released March 7, 2005.

Edelson, E. (2005) Even Mild Depression Ups Heart Failure Death Risk. www.healingwell.com . Retrieved on November 1, 2009 from http://news.healingwell.com/index.php?p=news1&id=524315

Gump, B. B., & Matthews, K. A. (2000). Are vacations good for your health?: The 9 year mortality experience after the multiple risk factor intervention trial. Psychosomatic Medicine, 62, 608-612.

Eaker, E. American Journal of Epidemiology, April 15, 1992; Vol. 135: pp 854-864.

www.livestrong.org